Case studies in psychopharmacology:

the use of drugs in psychiatry

.sea Psychiatylor
0170 Paton

MARTIN DUNITZ

© Martin Dunitz 1998

First published in the United Kingdom in 1998 by

Martin Dunitz Ltd
The Livery House
7–9 Pratt Street
London NW1 0AE

A CIP record for this book is available from the British Library.

ISBN 1-85317-653-2

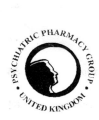

This publication is an approved text of the United Kingdom Psychiatric Pharmacy Group.

Printed and bound in Italy

Contents

Contributor List

Stephen Bazire BPharm MRPharmS
DipPsychPharm
Pharmacy Services Director
Norfolk Mental Health Care NHS Trust
Hellesdon Hospital
Norwich NR6 5BE
UK

David Branford PhD MRPharmS MCPP
Director of Pharmacy
Kingsway Hospital
Derby DE22 3LZ
UK

Jennie Day BSc MRPharmS MSc PhD
MRC Research Fellow
Department of Clinical Psychology
University of Liverpool
Liverpool L69 3BX
UK

John Donoghue BSc MRPharmS
Principal Pharmacist
Psychiatric Services
Wirral Hospital NHS Trust
Clatterbridge Hospital
Bebington
Wirral L63 4JY
UK

Denise Duncan BPharm DipClinPharm
MRPharmS
Senior Drug Information Pharmacist
Maudsley Hospital
Bethlem and Maudsley NHS Trust
London SE5 8AZ
UK

Celia L Feetam BPharm
MSc ACPP MRPharmS
Consultant Pharmacist
Wood Bond Priory Hospital
Birmingham B17 8BZ
UK

Ann Hutton BPharm MRPharmS
Clinical Pharmacist
Bethlem and Maudsley NHS Trust
Denmark Hill
London SE5 8AZ
UK

Robyn McAskill BPharm
DipClinPharm MRPharmS
Drug Information Pharmacist
Bethlem and Maudsley NHS Trust
Denmark Hill
London SE5 8AZ
UK

Shameem Mir BPharm DipPharmPrac
MRPharmS
Senior Clinical Pharmacist
Bethlem and Maudsley NHS Trust
Denmark Hill
London SE5 8AZ
UK

Carol Paton BSc DipClinPharm
MRPharmS
Principal Pharmacist
Oxleas NHS Trust
Bexley Hospital
Bexley, Kent DA5 2BW
UK

Peter Pratt BSc MRPharmS
Chief Pharmacist
Community Health Sheffield Trust
Lightwood House
Lightwood Lane
Sheffield S8 8BG
UK

Railton Scott BSc MSc MRPharmS RMN
Senior Clinical Pharmacist (Psychiatry)
Brighton Health Care NHS Trust
Brighton
UK

David Taylor BSc MSc MRPharmS
Chief Pharmacist/Honorary Senior
Lecturer
Institute of Psychiatry
Maudsley Hospital
Bethlem and Maudsley NHS Trust
London SE5 8AZ
UK

Preface

Almost all the drugs used in the treatment of psychiatric patients were discovered by accident (serendipity) 40 or more years ago. This has three consequences. First, the use of these drugs remained very empirical for many years; secondly, there were few adequately controlled studies concerning efficacy and safety; thirdly, these drugs have many unwanted and unnecessary side-effects. More recently, with the development of neuroscience, especially the discovery of receptors, more selective drugs have been developed. These have fewer side effects, although their efficacy, with the notable exception of clozapine, is largely unchanged. At the same time there have been many demands for evidence based medicine and this has been apparent in the field of psychopharmacology as well.

As a consequence, in large areas of drug treatment in psychiatry much more rational decisions can be made. Pharmacists have made a major contribution to these advances, carefully documenting those clinical trials that meet standards of adequacy, and even occasionally, of excellence. They are also assiduous in pointing out deficiencies in our knowledge.

It is accordingly a great pleasure for me to have been invited to write the preface to this unusual book. It comprises case histories in a variety of areas of clinical practice in psychiatry. These vignettes raise important questions concerning management. The various chapter authors, all pharmacists, then systematically review the available evidence. Where the evidence is still incomplete, they nevertheless attempt to provide reasonable management decisions to guide the day-to-day therapy of the patients. Pharmacokinetics is given prominence, as are the problems of polypharmacy. Copious references are included to guide the reader.

Thus both psychiatrists in training and those with extensive experience will find this book a mine of information on the evidence base for clinical psychopharmacology and drug treatment in psychiatry.

Malcolm Lader
OBE DSc PhD MD FRCPsych

Introduction

Psychopharmacology is an increasingly complex subject and one that has a growing influence on the treatment of mental illness. A knowledge of the intricacies of the clinical use of psychotropics is now essential to many of the professions involved in the treatment of the mentally ill. Despite this, there remain few reliable, up-to-date, comprehensive sources of information on the practical use of psychotropics.

This book, it is hoped, will fulfil an unmet need. It provides considered and well-supported advice on the use of psychotropics in common therapeutic areas encountered in psychiatric and general practice. Cases have been prepared by pharmacists working in psychiatry and who have a special interest in the subject covered in each case. The book includes consideration of all the information available to us at the end of March 1998. It is intended primarily to be a valuable resource for psychiatrists, junior doctors working in psychiatry, pharmacists and nurses. General practitioners and clinical psychologists may also find some or all of the cases useful in their practice.

David Taylor
Carol Paton
June 1998

Non-refractory schizophrenia

Carol Paton

SR, a 24-year-old Caucasian man, was brought to casualty by the police after being found wandering amongst the traffic on the local dual carriageway. He was agitated and perplexed, and exhibited poor self care. Rapport was poor and he muttered to himself around the themes of pollution, overcrowding and confusion. He admitted to second person auditory hallucinations instructing him to 'organise the streets' and third person auditory hallucinations which discussed his inability to do so. He exhibited formal thought disorder with knight's move thinking and described passivity phenomena.

SR had suffered from a psychotic episode 14 months previously which involved a three-month admission to hospital. He was treated with fluphenazine decanoate depot 50 mg every three weeks and procyclidine 5 mg three times a day and made a good recovery, returning to work in a hotel kitchen. He stopped his depot five months ago and has had no contact with services since.

SR had no significant medical history.

SR is the third of four siblings, had a normal birth and achieved normal early milestones, although later under- *achieved at secondary school. His paternal uncle had a diagnosis of schizophrenia and took his own life. Physical examination and blood tests were unremarkable and a urine drug screen was negative. The working diagnosis was that of a relapse of a schizophrenic illness.*

Questions

1. Describe and explain a typical pharmacological treatment algorithm for schizophrenia. Which drug would be appropriate in this case?
2. What are appropriate treatment doses of the commonly used antipsychotics?
3. What are the short- and long-term benefits of antipsychotics in schizophrenia? Quantify the risks of stopping treatment after recovery.
4. What are the short- and long-term risks of anticholinergics?

Answers

1. Describe and explain a typical pharmacological treatment algorithm for schizophrenia. Which drug would be appropriate in this case?

Most algorithms include, as the first step, a conventional antipsychotic such as haloperidol or trifluoperazine. If compliance is known or suspected to be a problem, and the patient is not neuroleptic naive, then a depot is appropriate early in treatment.

Antipsychotic efficacy is thought to be mediated through D2 blockade in the mesolimbic dopamine pathway in the brain. Conventional antipsychotics, through additional blockade of the nigrostriatal D2 pathway, cause extrapyramidal side-effects (EPSE) in a significant proportion of patients (American Psychiatric Association, 1997) ie acute dystonias in 10%, pseudoparkinsonism in 20%, akathisia (which has been linked to aggression and suicidal behaviour) in 20–25% and dysphoria (which is linked to non-compliance and subsequent poor outcome) in a significant proportion (King et al, 1995). Tardive dyskinesia, which can be irreversible, occurs at a rate of 4% per year of antipsychotic exposure (American Psychiatric Association, 1997). Procyclidine can be useful in the treatment of dystonias and pseudoparkinsonism, whereas propranolol or cyproheptadine are more useful in akathisia. Hyperprolactinaemia, due to blockade of the tuberoinfundibular D2 pathway, can result in galactorrhoea, amenorrhoea and gynaecomastia. Typical antipsychotics also cause, depending on their individual receptor-binding profiles, sedation (H1 block), postural hypotension (adrenergic alpha-1 block) and dry mouth, blurred vision, urinary retention and constipation (muscarinic block). Seizures and neuroleptic malignant syndrome can also occur.

There is little to be gained by substituting one typical drug for another, as a response rate of more than 5% is unlikely (Thompson, 1994). There is no objective evidence that combinations of antipsychotics offer any therapeutic advantage over single agents.

Treatment algorithms, therefore, usually indicate that, if any one typical antipsychotic is poorly tolerated or ineffective, an atypical drug should be tried. The term 'atypical' was originally associated with the inability of a compound to produce catalepsy in laboratory animals (a screening model thought to have good predictive validity in identifying potential antipsychotic agents). Atypical antipsychotics have also been variously defined as having no effect on serum prolactin, improved efficacy against negative symptoms, being highly selective D2 blockers (eg pimozide) or relatively selective for D2 receptors in mesolimbic areas (eg the withdrawn agent, remoxipride), having a high 5HT2 : D2 receptor blocking ratio (eg risperidone, olanzapine) or high intrinsic anticholinergic activity (eg thioridazine). The lack of an accepted standard definition should make it immediately apparent that all atypicals are not the same. Many consider the only true atypical to be clozapine, which is discussed in the chapter on treatment-resistant schizophrenia. For the purposes of this discussion only the recently introduced antipsychotics, risperidone, sertindole, olanzapine, quetiapine and amisulpride along with sulpiride will be considered broadly to fit the definition of atypicality.

Sulpiride is associated with fewer EPSE than conventional antipsychotics, but raises serum prolactin. It is available only as a liquid or a 200-mg tablet, sometimes making it necessary for a large number of tablets to be taken each day (licensed maximum 12).

Of the newer drugs, risperidone has been shown in good, double-blind, placebo-controlled trials to be an effective antipsychotic at a dose of 6 mg per day, although it raises prolactin levels and doses above 8 mg per day are associated with an increased incidence of EPSEs (Chouinard et al, 1993).

Sertindole is relatively selective for mesolimbic D2 receptors (at least in animals), requires dosage titration (due to alpha-1 adrenergic effects) and has little effect on prolactin, but prolongs the QTc interval, making ECG monitoring essential. Sertindole also interacts with many other drugs; SSRIs, tricyclics, ketoconazole and erythromycin can all inhibit the metabolism of sertindole, thus potentially raising serum levels and increasing the risk of QTc prolongation. In addition, sertindole should not be given with drugs that can potentially cause electrolyte disturbances such as diuretics, or to patients with pre-existing cardiac pathology. Olanzapine produces very few EPSEs and only a transient rise in prolactin. Transient rises in LFTs can occur early in treatment. In a multicentre trial involving 1996 patients, olanzapine was shown to have superior overall antipsychotic efficacy to haloperidol (Tollefson et al, 1997). It must be emphasised that the patients included in this trial were not selected for previous treatment resistance, and there is currently no objective evidence that olanzapine is effective in this group of patients.

Quetiapine has a similar profile to sertindole in that it has no effect on prolactin, a very low ('placebo level') incidence of EPSEs and dosage titration is required.

Amisulpride is structurally related to sulpiride and shares its low propensity to cause EPSEs and potent prolactin-elevating effects.

While this group of drugs produce significantly fewer dopamine-mediated side-effects than the conventional antipsychotics, side-effects due to blockade of other receptors do occur. For example, olanzapine has anticholinergic side-effects and is sedative; risperidone and sertindole cause postural hypotension significant enough to require that the dose be increased slowly at the start of treatment.

There are arguments in favour of using atypicals first line (Kerwin, 1996), particularly in first-episode schizophrenia, where it is hoped that improved tolerability will lead to an improvement in long-term compliance, and therefore outcome, although not all would subscribe to this view (Barnes, 1996). Objective data in this area are lacking, although a recent study demonstrated that treatment with risperidone led to a higher subjective quality of life than treatment with conventional antipsychotics (Franz et al, 1997). The large cost differential (haloperidol 10 mg = £7.80/month, risperidone 6 mg = £117/month), however, makes the first-line use of atypicals for all psychotic patients untenable for the majority of units. Discussion of the algorithm further than this point for the 30% of patients who are 'treatment resistant' is covered in the chapter on treatment-resistant schizophrenia.

The patient in this case previously made a good recovery with fluphenazine depot 50 mg every three weeks. His reason for discontinuing treatment is unclear. If side-effects were not the reason, fluphenazine should be prescribed again. Otherwise an atypical drug should be prescribed as monotherapy with sedative cover, if required early in treatment, provided by a benzodiazepine.

2. What are appropriate treatment doses of the commonly used antipsychotics?
Although therapeutic doses are more clearly defined for the newer antipsychotics, data for the older drugs do exist. Rifkin et al (1991) randomly assigned 87 new admissions with schizophrenia to receive 10, 30 or 80 mg of haloperidol daily and followed them over an eight-week period. The higher doses had no advantage over the 10 mg dose in either speed or magnitude of response.

The optimum dose for risperidone is 4–8 mg per day with higher doses leading to an increased incidence of EPSE (Chouinard et al, 1993) which negates the major advantage that risperidone holds over the older drugs. Risperidone is licensed up to a daily maximum dose of 16 mg and prescribers are more aware of this licensed maximum dose than the clinical efficacy data. Poor prescribing practice in this area was highlighted by a recent large survey of risperidone prescribing (Taylor et al, 1997) which found that only 15% of patients prescribed risperidone received it as the sole antipsychotic at a dose of 8 mg or less each day, without concurrent anticholinergics.

Chlorpromazine 400–1000 mg per day and olanzapine 10–20 mg per day have also been shown to be therapeutic daily doses in the majority of patients (American Psychiatric Association, 1997). High (above BNF maxima) doses of antipsychotics are probably of little benefit to the majority of patients who receive them, and are associated with significant risks. This area is reviewed in detail in the Royal College of Psychiatrists Consensus Statement on the use of high-dose antipsychotics (Thompson, 1994). This paper is essential reading for all practising psychiatrists.

Care should be taken not to confuse the non-specific sedation that many antipsychotics produce with actual antipsychotic effect. Sedation, if required early in treatment, should be provided by a sedative (usually a benzodiazepine, which can be withdrawn when no longer required) rather than as the side-effect of an antipsychotic.

3. What are the short- and long-term benefits of antipsychotics in schizophrenia? Quantify the risks of stopping treatment after recovery.

In the short term, antipsychotics control behaviour and improve the positive and negative symptoms of schizophrenia. There are good objective data to show that the more rapidly psychosis is treated, the more favourable is the long-term outcome (Szymanski et al, 1996). Sixty per cent of antipsychotic-treated patients (as compared with 20% who receive placebo) have been shown to improve significantly over a six-week period (American Psychiatric Association, 1997). Although an important part of the therapeutic benefit occurs in this time span (Keck et al, 1989), improvements in socialisation can continue for many months.

Many double-blind, placebo-controlled trials have demonstrated the benefits of antipsychotics in the maintenance phase of schizophrenia. In a summary of data involving 3609 patients, 20% of those who were maintained on active medication relapsed as compared with 53% of those who were maintained on placebo (Kaplin & Sadcock, 1989). In a review of 66 studies on antipsychotic withdrawal involving 4365 patients who were followed up for a mean of 9.7 months, over three times as many patients withdrawn from antipsychotics (53%) relapsed compared to those who remained on maintenance treatment (16%) (Gilbert et al, 1995). The many studies that are reviewed in this paper lead to the conclusion that the shorter the symptom-free period and the longer the duration of follow-up, the more likely is relapse.

Relapse has been shown to be more likely after abrupt rather than gradual discontinuation of oral antipsychotics (Viguera et al, 1997), with depot antipsychotics offering a similar protective effect, probably because of the slow elimination of active drug from the body.

Evidence from primary research, as well as from consensus opinions of expert groups (Kissling et al, 1991), indicates that first-episode patients should be treated with antipsychotics for at least one to two years and multi-episode patients for at least five years.

The patient in this case has had two episodes of illness in a 14-month period. Relapse followed five months after his depot was stopped. He is at high risk of further episodes if he does not comply with maintenance antipsychotic treatment.

4. What are the short- and long-term risks of anticholinergics?

Anticholinergics can cause dry mouth, blurred vision, constipation, urinary retention and tachycardia. Higher doses can cause confusion, particularly in the elderly. Some patients feel subjectively better when taking anticholinergics and, in a minority, they are misused for their euphoric effects.

Anticholinergics worsen existing tardive dyskinesia (TD) (Greil et al, 1985), but there is little objective evidence to support anticholinergics as an independent risk factor for TD (Gardos & Cole, 1983). Anticholinergics are more likely to be prescribed for those patients who experience EPSEs early in treatment, a group who are known to be more likely to develop TD. It has been suggested that the use of anticholinergics in these patients is coincidental to the development of TD, rather than being directly responsible (a so-called epiphenomenon) (Barnes, 1990).

Key points

- The more rapidly psychosis is treated, the more favourable the long-term outcome.
- Non-specific sedation should not be confused with antipsychotic effect.
- There is good evidence to suggest that the doses of antipsychotics

routinely used in clinical practice are too high.

- Atypical antipsychotics cause less severe EPSEs than the older drugs, but are much more expensive.
- Individual antipsychotics have different side-effect profiles.
- Most treatment algorithms recommend a typical drug followed by an atypical followed by clozapine.
- First-episode patients should be treated for one to two years, multi-episode patients for at least five years.
- Relapse is less likely after discontinuation of depot or slow reduction of oral therapy, than after abrupt withdrawal of oral antipsychotics.
- The relapse rate within one to two years is three times higher in those who stop treatment compared with those who continue to take antipsychotics.

References

American Psychiatric Association (1997) Practice guidelines for the treatment of patients with schizophrenia, *Am J Psychiatry* **154:**4 (suppl) 1–49.

Barnes TRE (1990) Comment on the WHO consensus statement, *Br J Psychiatry* **156:** 413–14.

Barnes TRE (1996) Commentary: Response to Professor Kerwin, *Psychiatr Bull* **20:** 26–9.

Chouinard G, Jones B, Remington G et al (1993) A Canadian multi-centre placebo controlled study of fixed doses of risperidone and haloperidol in the treatment of chronic schizophrenia patients, *J Clin Psychopharmacol* **13:**(1) 25–40.

Franz M, Lis S, Pludderman K et al (1997) Conventional versus atypical neuroleptics: subjective quality of life in schizophrenia patients, *Br J Psychiatry* **170:** 422–5.

Gardos G, Cole JD (1983) Tardive dyskinesia and anticholinergic drugs, *Am J Psychiatry* **140:** 200–2.

Gilbert PL, Harris MJ, McAdams LA et al (1995) Neuroleptic withdrawal in schizophrenia patients. A review of the literature, *Arch Gen Psychiatry* **52:** 173–88.

Greil W, Haag H, Rossnagl G et al (1985) Effect of anticholinergics on tardive dyskinesia: a controlled study, *Br J Psychiatry* **145:** 304–10.

Kaplin HI, Sadcock BJ (eds) (1989) *Comprehensive Textbook of Psychiatry*, 5th edn, vol 2. (Baltimore MD: Williams & Wiltkins) 1607.

Keck P, Cohen B, Baldessanni R et al (1989) Time course of antipsychotic effects on neuroleptic drugs, *Am J Psychiatry* **146:** 1289–92.

Kerwin R (1996) An essay on the use of new antipsychotics, *Psychiatr Bull* **20:** 23–9.

King DJ, Burke M, Lucas RA (1995) Antipsychotic drug induced dysphoria, *Br J Psychiatry* **167:** 480–2.

Kissling W, Kane JM, Barnes SJ et al (1991) Guidelines for neuroleptic relapse prevention in schizophrenia: towards a consensus review. In: Kissling WW, ed. *Schizophrenia* (Berlin: Springer-Verlag) 155–63.

Rifkin A, Doddi S, Karajgi B et al (1991) Dosage of haloperidol for schizophrenia, *Arch Gen Psychiatry* **48:** 166–70.

Szymanski SR, Cannon TT, Gallagher F et al (1996) Course of treatment response in first episode and chronic schizophrenia, *Am J Psychiatry* **153:** 519–25.

Taylor D, Holmes R, Hilton T et al (1997) Evaluating and improving the quality of risperidone prescribing, *Psychiatr Bull* **21:** 680–3.

Thompson C for the Royal College of Psychiatrists consensus panel (1994) Consensus statement on the use of high dose antipsychotic medication, *Br J Psychiatry* **164:** 448–58.

Tollefson GD, Beasley CM, Tran PV et al (1997) Olanzapine versus haloperidol in the treatment of schizophrenia and schizoaffective and schizophreniform disorders: results of an international collaborative trial, *Am J Psychiatry* **154:** 457–65.

Viguera AC, Baldessarini RJ, Hegerty JD et al (1997) Clinical risk following abrupt and gradual withdrawal of maintenance neuroleptic treatment, *Arch Gen Psychiatry* **54:** 49–55.

Recommended Further Reading

Tardive Dyskinesia: A task force report of the American Psychiatric Association. American Psychiatric Association, Washington, 1992.

Refractory schizophrenia

David Taylor

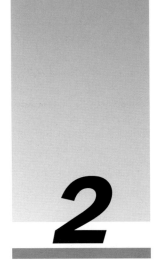

SK is a 26-year-old Iranian man with a five-year history of psychotic illness. His first episode was treated in Iran with trifluoperazine, prochlorperazine and sulpiride in combination. Clinical details are scant, but it appears that he recovered well and was discharged from hospital after three weeks.

SK later came to the UK and was soon admitted with marked delusions, auditory hallucinations and thought disorder with neologisms. He responded to chlorpromazine 600 mg per day and was discharged. A diagnosis of paranoid schizophrenia was made.

SK was referred to a specialist psychosis unit following poor recent response to a range of antipsychotics (trifluoperazine 60 mg per day; haloperidol 40 mg per day; zuclopenthixol depot 600 mg per week). He admitted to hearing voices telling him to 'smoke' (he chain-smokes 50+ cigarettes a day) and to 'hit-out', and was profoundly suspicious of other patients. SK appeared lethargic with no arm swinging on walking and a slow monotone voice. His medication on referral was as follows:

Risperidone	3 mg BD
Carbamazepine	300 mg BD
Clonazepam	2 mg ON
Thioridazine	100 mg at night

Questions

1. What is the drug of choice in this patient?
2. What is the evidence supporting the use of new atypical antipsychotics in refractory schizophrenia?
3. How is clozapine therapy optimised?
4. How are adverse effects managed?

Answers

1. What is the drug of choice in this patient?

SK is evidently suffering from schizophrenia which is refractory to treatment. Clozapine is the only drug shown unequivocally to be effective in refractory schizophrenia and it is therefore the drug of choice in SK.

Evidence of the efficacy of clozapine in refractory schizophrenia derives largely from the seminal study of Kane et al (1988). Subjects in this study were defined as treatment-resistant: each had received at least three antipsychotics at high dose for six weeks and had not responded. All were severely ill with a Brief Psychiatric Rating Scale (scored 1–7) score (BPRS) of at least 45. In a single-blind run-in period, all subjects received high-dose haloperidol to ensure treatment-resistance (1.6% of subjects responded). Subjects then received either clozapine (up to 900 mg per day) or chlorpromazine (up to 1800 mg per day). After six weeks, 30% of clozapine-treated patients had responded (>20% fall in BPRS and final score of <35) compared with 4% of the chlorpromazine-treated group.

Other studies have shown that response rates with clozapine are higher than 60% if the drug is given for up to a year (Meltzer et al, 1989; Conley et al, 1997). All patients should therefore receive at least a six-month trial of clozapine to assess its effectiveness properly.

In the case of SK, clozapine should be introduced as early as possible. Carbamazepine should be withdrawn gradually before clozapine is started. Assuming a normal full blood count, risperidone and thioridazine may be slowly withdrawn once clozapine has been initiated (Taylor, 1997a), although risperidone can increase clozapine plasma levels (Taylor, 1997b). It should be noted that SK is a heavy smoker. Cigarette smoke induces the hepatic metabolising enzyme CPY1A2, which is involved in the metabolism of clozapine (Taylor, 1997b). SK may, therefore, eventually require a higher than average dose of clozapine.

2. What is the evidence supporting the use of new atypical antipsychotics in refractory schizophrenia?
This is a subject of some debate and one in which assumption, misunderstanding and misinformation greatly influence clinical practice.

Clozapine was the first drug to be termed 'atypical', essentially because it was observed not to cause acute

extrapyramidal adverse effects or to cause catelepsy in rats. It is also unarguably effective in refractory schizophrenia. The mechanism by which clozapine exerts its superior antipsychotic effect is not understood. All atypical antipsychotics have different receptor binding profiles, with clozapine being a particularly 'dirty drug'. Firm associations between receptor activity and clinical effects have, in many cases, not been made. Therefore, lack of EPSE and efficacy in refractory illness cannot be assumed to be directly linked. Nevertheless, many clinicians now assume that any new drug to which the label atypical is applied has similar efficacy to clozapine. New atypicals are widely used in refractory schizophrenia. However, evidence supporting their use in this condition is weak.

Risperidone has been closely evaluated in refractory schizophrenia, but virtually no useful information has emerged. Bondolfi and co-workers' much-cited study (Bondolfi et al, 1995) is claimed to demonstrate that risperidone and clozapine have equal efficacy in 'treatment-resistant, chronic schizophrenia'. Criticisms of the report include the following (the list is not exhaustive):

- Some subjects were treatment-intolerant, not treatment-refractory. (Proportions not specified.)
- Clozapine was increased to 300 mg/day over seven days (so adversely affecting tolerability).
- Mean clozapine dose at end point was only 291.2 mg/day.
- Response rates were remarkably high (>60%).
- Many methodological details are not described (run-in period, previous therapy, assessor details, power calculations, statistical tests used, etc).

This abstract should be viewed with these observations in mind.

Experience from clinical practice strongly suggests that risperidone has very limited efficacy in truly refractory schizophrenia. In addition, switching from clozapine to risperidone seems largely disastrous (Lacey et al, 1995) and, as Reus (1997) has observed, if risperidone were really as effective as clozapine, than it would have rapidly supplanted the more toxic drug. It has not, and clozapine remains the drug of choice for refractory schizophrenia.

Very little information is available on the other, new atypical drugs.

Sertindole has not been formally evaluated in treatment-refractory schizophrenia and its manufacturers do not promote its use in such patients.

Olanzapine is chemically and pharmacologically similar to clozapine, so some similarity in efficacy might be expected. In the large trial of Tollefson et al (1997), the authors consider that their data 'provide a signal that olanzapine offers potential in the treatment of non-responders' (to previous neuroleptic treatment). While their data do show that olanzapine offers important advantages over haloperidol, it is wrong to extrapolate these findings and to infer any special efficacy in refractory illness: subjects had mild illness and many were treatment-intolerant. A more recent naturalistic study of 56 patients (Taylor et al, 1998) has shown that, in severe, treatment-refractory psychosis, the response rate with olanzapine after six weeks was nil. A similar, open, uncontrolled study (Martin et al, 1997) produced rather different results, with 36% of refractory patients responding to olanzapine 15–25 mg/day. Indeed, it has been suggested that higher doses of olanzapine (e.g. up to and above 40 mg/day) might be effective in refractory patients. However, extrapyramidal side-effects are common at high doses (Sheitman et al, 1997). The costs of such a treatment regime are also prohibitive (around £5,000 per patient per year).

Quetiapine, amisulpride and ziprasidone have not been formally studied in refractory schizophrenia.

Thus, there is essentially no cogent evidence supporting the use of new atypical drugs in refractory schizophrenia. Clozapine remains the drug of choice and should continue to be so until compelling evidence to the contrary emerges from well-conducted, scientifically robust clinical trials.

3. How is clozapine therapy optimised?

Clozapine is introduced at 12.5 mg at night and the dose increased over two to three weeks. For most patients a dose of 400 mg a day is aimed for, at least initially. Further increases up to a maximum of 900 mg/day may be necessary. It is common to use increments of 50 mg/day perhaps every two weeks, based on careful evaluation. Recognised clinical rating scales such as the BPRS and the Clinical Global Impression are helpful in measuring change and provide a useful, meaningful record of drug response.

Many centres use plasma level monitoring to optimise clozapine dose. Plasma levels above 350 µg/l are usually associated with response (Taylor and Duncan, 1995) although this threshold level should be considered simply as a guide: many patients respond with lower levels and some fail to respond despite higher levels. Plasma level determinations are also invaluable in revealing occult non-compliance; a rare but significant problem even with inpatients. They can also help identify patients with high clearance rates and sub-therapeutic levels (usually male smokers). Dangerous pharmacokinetic interactions (Taylor, 1997b) can also be closely monitored.

Once dose and plasma level have been optimised, clozapine should be given for a lengthy period to evaluate response. How long this evaluation period should be is the subject of some debate. Meltzer et al (1989) showed that clinical response to clozapine was delayed in many patients with some not reaching a predetermined threshold for response for six or nine months. A year-long trial period thus became standard with clinicians noting continued improvement even beyond this time. However, this practice has been challenged (Carpenter et al, 1995) on the basis that patients do not suddenly begin to improve after many months, but do so gradually (but noticeably), reaching a somewhat arbitrary threshold for response after many months. An assessment period of two to four months was suggested, with patients showing 'little or no benefit' during this time being recommended for withdrawal. This view, in turn, was robustly challenged (Meltzer, 1995) and so the debate has continued. More recently Conley et al (1997) have contributed to this debate with the observation that all responders meet response criteria within eight weeks of a change in dose. Thus there seems little point in continuing with a given dose of clozapine beyond this time. It was also noted that dose titration to 600 mg/day over 12–18 weeks identified 90% of responders. Plasma level monitoring was not used.

Taken together, these observations and arguments provide clinicians with little in the way of clear, practical guidance. Perhaps the best that can be concluded is as follows:

- Begin clozapine and slowly increase to 400 mg/day over two to three weeks, or longer if necessary.

- If no response is observed over several weeks at 400 mg/day, then the dose should be adjusted to afford a plasma level of more than 350 µg/l.
- If no response is observed (again over several weeks), the dose should be increased to the maximum tolerated dose.
- If no response is observed after eight weeks at the maximum tolerated dose, then clozapine should be withdrawn.

In practice, these guidelines will usually result in trial periods of four to six months overall. Predetermined criteria for response should be drawn up locally. A 20% fall in Brief Psychiatric Rating Scale score is a widely accepted criterion for useful clinical improvement, but overall quality of life is also an important consideration. The co-administration of other antipsychotics should be avoided. A possible exception to this is low-dose sulpiride, which may be effective in clozapine partial responders (Shiloh et al, 1997). However, this trial should be interpreted with caution, as the cohorts randomised to receive clozapine and placebo had significantly different baseline scores on some items, indicating that they may have been a more chronically ill group than those randomised to receive clozapine and sulpiride. Also, patient numbers were low.

4. How are adverse effects managed?
The most serious adverse effects of clozapine are neutropenia and agranulocytosis which are well managed by the Clozaril Patient Monitoring Service run by Novartis (Atkin et al, 1996). These potentially fatal adverse effects should be considered the only adverse effects serious enough to warrant discontinuation of clozapine. All other adverse effects eventually abate or can be successfully managed with remedial therapies.

Drowsiness can be severe but this wears off after three to six months at the most. Giving a larger proportion of the total daily dose at night often helps. **Constipation** is common but responds to stimulant (e.g. senna) and bulk forming (e.g. ispaghula) laxatives in combination. **Hypersalivation** is also common but may be effectively treated by hyoscine 300–600 µg at night or pirenzepine 25–100 mg/day (Fritze and Elliger, 1995).
Hypotension is usually relieved by reducing the dose of clozapine or slowing the rate of increase. In severe, dose-limiting cases, moclobemide in combination with Bovril is helpful

(Taylor et al, 1995). **Hypertension** occurs less often and can be successfully treated with propranolol (George and Winther, 1996).

Weight gain is very common (Bustillo et al, 1996) and difficult to prevent or treat. Dietary counselling would seem a sensible precaution but there are no firm data on its effectiveness.

Nocturnal enuresis is rare but often troublesome when it does occur. Avoiding late evening fluids is helpful and desmopressin can be used in severe cases (Aponowitz et al, 1995).

Seizures occur at high doses (Wilson and Claussen, 1994) but are effectively prevented by co-administration of therapeutic doses (plasma levels 50–100 mg/l) of valproate.

Nausea is quite common but generally short-lived.

Key points

- Clozapine is the drug of choice for treatment refractory schizophrenia.
- There is no good objective evidence demonstrating the efficacy of other atypical antipsychotics in treatment-refractory schizophrenia.

- Serum-level monitoring may be useful in optimising clozapine treatment, aiming for levels of above 350 μg/l.
- If no response is shown to the maximum tolerated dose administered for eight weeks, clozapine should be withdrawn.
- Agranulocytosis is the most serious side-effect of clozapine. This risk is managed safely by the CPMS.
- Drowsiness, constipation, hypersalivation, nocturnal enuresis and seizures can all occur, but can be managed. Symptomatic postural hypotension and weight gain are more difficult to manage.

References

Aponowitz JS, Safferman AZ, Lieberman JA (1995) Management of clozapine-induced enuresis, *Am J Psychiatry* **152:** 472.

Atkin F, Kendall F, Gould D et al (1996) Neutropenia and agranulocytosis in patients receiving clozapine in the UK and Ireland, *Br J Psychiatry* **169:** 483–8.

Bondolfi G, Baumann P, Patris M et al (1995) A randomised double-blind trial of risperidone versus clozapine for treatment-resistant chronic schizophrenia. Abstract from *8th ECNP Congress*, Venice, Italy, October 1995.

Bustillo JR, Buchanan RW, Irish D et al (1996) Differential effect of clozapine on weight: a controlled study, *Am J Psychiatry* **153:** 817–19.

Carpenter WT Jr, Conley RR, Buchanan RW et al (1995) Patient response and resource management: another view of clozapine treatment of schizophrenia, *Am J Psychiatry* **152:** 827.

Conley RR, Carpenter WT, Tamminga CA (1997) Time to clozapine response in a standardized trial, *Am J Psychiatry* **154:** 1243–7.

Fritze J, Elliger T (1995) Pirenzepine for clozapine-induced hypersalivation, *Lancet* **346:** 1034.

George TP, Winther LC (1996) Hypertension after initiation of clozapine, *Am J Psychiatry* **153:** 1368–9.

Kane J, Honifeld G, Singer J et al (1988) Clozapine for the treatment-resistant schizophrenia, *Arch Gen Psychiatry* **45:** 789–96.

Lacey RL, Preskorn SH, Jerkovich GS (1995) Is risperidone a substitute for clozapine for patients who do not respond to neuroleptics? *Am J Psychiatry* **152:** 1401.

Martin J, Gomez J-C, Garcia-Bernardo E et al (1997) Olanzapine in treatment-refractory schizophrenia: results of an open-label study, *J Clin Psychiatry* **58:** 479–83.

Meltzer HY (1995) Clozapine: is another view valid? *Am J Psychiatry* **152:** 821–5.

Meltzer HY, Bastani B, Young Kwon K et al (1989) A prospective study of clozapine in treatment-resistant schizophrenic patients. *Psychopharmacology* **99:** 568–72.

Reus VI (1997) Olanzapine, *Lancet* **350:** 594.

Sheitman BB, Lindgren JC, Early J, Sved M (1997) High-dose olanzapine for treatment-refractory schizophrenia, *Am J Psychiatry* **154:** 1626.

Shiloh R, Zemishlany Z, Aizenberg D et al (1997) Sulpiride augmentation in people with schizophrenia partially responsive to clozapine: a double-blind, placebo-controlled study, *Br J Psychiatry* **171:** 569–73.

Taylor D (1997a) Switching from typical to atypical antipsychotics: practical guidelines, *CNS Drugs* **8:** 285–91.

Taylor D (1997b) Pharmacokinetic interactions involving clozapine, *Br J Psychiatry* **171:** 109–12.

Taylor D, Duncan D (1995) The use of clozapine plasma levels in optimising therapy, *Psychiatr Bull* **19:** 753–5.

Taylor D, Mir S, Mace S (1998) Olanzapine in practice – a naturalistic study, *Acta Psych Scand*, submitted.

Taylor D, Reveley A, Faivre F (1995) Clozapine-induced hypotension treated with moclobemide and Bovril, *Br J Psychiatry* **167:** 409–10.

Tollefson GD, Tran PV, Street JS et al (1997) Olanzapine versus haloperidol in the treatment of schizophrenia and schizoaffective and schizophreniform disorders: results of an international collaborative trial, *Am J Psychiatry* **154:** 457–65.

Wilson WH, Claussen AM (1994) Seizures associated with clozapine treatment in a state hospital, *J Clin Psychiatry* **55:** 184–8.

Clozapine use in the elderly

John Donoghue

3

DF, a 71-year-old woman with a diagnosis of schizoaffective disorder and a 30-year history of mental illness, was admitted to hospital from a nursing home, with a presenting history of deterioration in her mental state over the past two weeks. Staff at the home reported that she had been throwing herself onto the floor and refusing to get up, and responding to second person auditory hallucinations telling her to hurt herself by burning her face with cigarettes. She was experiencing persecutory delusions and had been aggressive.

On admission DF was uncooperative and agitated and seemed unaware of her surroundings and people in her vicinity. She also appeared preoccupied by auditory hallucinations and did not answer questions that were put to her. Her appearance was unkempt, she looked tired and had pronounced orofacial dyskinetic movements.

Her medication on admission was:

Carbamazepine SR	400 mg	nocte
Flupenthixol depot	100 mg	2 weekly
Trifluoperazine	20 mg	tds
Chlorpromazine	100 mg	8 am and 2 pm
Chlorpromazine	200 mg	nocte
Procyclidine	5 mg	qid
Lactulose	10 ml	bd
Senna	One tablet	nocte
Co-Codamol	Two tablets	qid prn
Nitrazepam	10 mg	nocte

After one week on the ward, DF showed no sign of improvement. She continued to throw herself onto the floor and reported voices saying:

'Two eyes in the sky see you're no good you bitch!'
'We're going to pull your eyes out.'
'She's dead already.'

DF appeared disorientated and refused to co-operate with even simple requests. Left to her own devices, she paced endlessly up and down corridors.

Her carbamazepine level was reported as 1 mg/l (12 hours post-dose).

Investigation for a urinary tract infection was negative.

There was no other significant medical history. Routine blood tests were normal.

After one month, the situation has changed little. DF attacked a fellow patient and, when staff tried to intervene, she broke a glass and attempted to stab the staff member with it. She was transferred to the intensive therapy ward where she refused to leave her room. DF removed her clothes and lay on her bed, curled in a fetal position, staring at the wall. It was decided to prescribe clozapine as the next step, because response to typical drugs had been poor.

Questions

1. Discuss the efficacy and tolerability of clozapine in the elderly, with particular reference to DF.
2. Which medicines should be discontinued in this patient before clozapine is started?
3. If no improvement was immediately apparent, how long should clozapine be continued before it is decided that it has not been effective?
4. What psychiatric complications might DF face if clozapine treatment has to be discontinued abruptly?
5. What evidence is there that clozapine may be beneficial in reducing symptoms of tardive dyskinesia?

Answers

1. Discuss the efficacy and tolerability of clozapine in the elderly, with particular reference to DF.

Clozapine is indicated for patients with treatment-refractory schizophrenia, or for those who are intolerant of conventional antipsychotic agents because of extrapyramidal effects, including tardive dyskinesia (Lieberman et al, 1989).

Operationally, the criteria for defining treatment resistance are that the patient should have failed to respond to full treatment doses of two antipsychotic agents of different classes given for adequate periods of time.

Superficially, this appears to have been the case with DF. Moreover, she appears to have developed a marked tardive dyskinesia. Note, however, that compliance with drug therapy may have been poor. This is indicated by low plasma levels of carbamazepine on admission.

DF is receiving relatively high doses of combined antipsychotic treatment. This may be associated with a worsening of symptoms and behaviour. Some of her problems may stem from akathisia, which has been linked to aggression (Schulk, 1985), or mental dulling resulting from the combination of medication she receives. There is virtually no firm evidence to support such treatment strategies (Thompson, 1994).

To determine whether DF meets the criteria for the use of clozapine, a full drug history should be taken. Even then, before clozapine is started, reduction in the numbers of antipsychotic agents currently prescribed and their doses should be attempted to see if there is an improved response to lower doses. Preferably, all antipsychotics should be withdrawn before clozapine is started (Taylor, 1997a).

In this patient, clozapine may have a superior antipsychotic effect and may lead to an improvement in tardive dyskinesia (Lieberman et al, 1991), a reduction in violence (Ratey et al, 1993) and a greatly simplified medication regimen. Clozapine also has beneficial effects on mood (Meltzer et al, 1995). However, the use of clozapine has not been investigated systematically in the elderly, although a few series of case reports have been published (Chengappa et al, 1995; Frankenburg and Kalunion, 1994).

Interestingly, different authors use different cut-off points when describing 'elderly' patients. Frankenburg and Kalunion (1994), for example, described a series of eight patients aged over 65, with a variety of diagnoses (psychotic depression, organic delusional disorder and schizophrenia). Two patients also had Parkinson's disease. Six of these patients were considered to have responded to clozapine at daily doses of between 12.5 and 400 mg although sedation, confusion and orthostatic hypotension were considered to be more problematic than in younger adults. Chenagappa et al (1995) described a further series of 12 patients, this time over 60 years of age. Seven of these patients suffered from clozapine-related postural hypotension. It was noted that slow dosage titration improved tolerability in this cohort. The observation that older patients may be at increased risk of a variety of adverse effects has been confirmed by Herst and Powell (1997).

The elderly often have reduced cardiac, hepatic and renal function. They also have a lower body water content and increased body fat. In general, the elderly will have greater problems with adverse drug reactions. Concern has been expressed that older, especially female, patients will be at increased risk of agranulocytosis (Alvir et al, 1993; Herst and Powell, 1997).

Clozapine is an alpha receptor antagonist, so postural hypotension is a common problem; and likely to be worse in elderly patients with decreased cardiac output. There may also be problems with drug interactions. The elderly have a greater degree of physical ill health and are more likely to be co-prescribed medicines likely to interact with clozapine.

Hypotensive effects can be minimised by starting at a low dose of clozapine (12.5 mg daily) and titrating doses more slowly than usual, over a period of four to six weeks, monitoring blood pressure regularly. It may be possible that a therapeutic effect is achieved with lower doses in the elderly, so responses should be carefully monitored to ensure that doses are not increased unnecessarily. Many patients are adequately treated with 100–200 mg daily. Co-prescribed medicines should be kept to a minimum, especially medicines that are hypotensive or sedative, and close attention should be paid to the possible development of agranulocytosis (Chengappa et al, 1995) or pharmacokinetic interactions (Taylor, 1997b).

DF has no significant physical pathology and has tolerated large doses of conventional antipsychotics. There is, therefore, no reason other than those already mentioned to suspect that DF will fail to tolerate clozapine.

2. Which medicines should be discontinued in this patient before clozapine is started?
Other drugs that have the potential to suppress the bone marrow should not be prescribed with clozapine. In the case of DF, this includes carbamazepine, trifluoperazine and chlorpromazine. Similarly, depot antipsychotics should not be administered with clozapine. As well as being pharmacologically illogical, it is thought that the presence of a depot may significantly impair the speed at which the bone marrow can recover should clozapine-induced agranulocytosis occur. Procyclidine, which may be exacerbating DF's tardive dyskinesia, is unlikely to be required when clozapine therapy is established. It will also contribute to the anticholinergic load produced by clozapine, with all the associated side-effects. Benzodiazepines should not be administered with clozapine, particularly during the period of clozapine dosage titration, as an interaction between the two resulting in severe sedation, hypersalivation, hypotension, toxic delirium, collapse, loss of consciousness and respiratory arrest

has been reported (Grohmann et al, 1989; Cobb et al, 1991).

DF is acutely disturbed and the transfer to clozapine may be problematic. Skilled nursing care in the psychiatric Intensive Therapy Unit (ITU) will be essential. While clozapine is being introduced, droperidol may be used to provide a calming effect, but only as a short-term measure.

3. If no improvement was immediately apparent, how long should clozapine be continued before it is decided that it has not been effective?

There are no data from controlled trials to indicate a minimum trial period for clozapine in the elderly. It would appear prudent to follow guidelines that exist for treatment with younger patients (Sajatovic et al, 1997).

4. What psychiatric complications might DF face if clozapine treatment has to be discontinued abruptly?

A clozapine withdrawal syndrome consisting of severe psychotic relapse in addition to agitation, restlessness, confusion, sweating and aggression has been reported by Palia and Clarke (1993). Supersensitivity psychosis has also been reported (Ekblom et al, 1984) as has rebound psychosis (Parsa

et al, 1993). The emergent psychotic symptoms are often refractory to treatment. As the majority of patients treated with clozapine have treatment-refractory schizophrenia, reports of the emergence of psychotic symptoms refractory to treatment with other neuroleptics after sudden clozapine withdrawal should be interpreted carefully.

5. What evidence is there that clozapine may be beneficial in reducing symptoms of tardive dyskinesia?

There is a possbility that clozapine may reduce the symptoms of tardive dyskinesia experienced by this patient. A review of published studies of the effect of clozapine on tardive dyskinesia concluded that approximately 43% of patients could experience at least a 50% reduction in symptoms (Lieberman et al, 1991).

However, this conclusion must be regarded as tentative as there were methodological limitations in the studies reviewed which made comparisons between them difficult. It appears that patients with dystonic movements rather than choreoathetoid movements are more likely to benefit. These findings await confirmation by controlled trials.

Key points

- Clozapine is probably an effective treatment for refractory psychosis in the elderly.
- Sedation, confusion, orthostatic hypotension and agranulocytosis may occur more frequently and be more troublesome than in younger adults.
- Slow upward dosage titration improves tolerability and gives the best chance of success. Much lower doses than those required by younger adults may be effective.
- Particular care must be taken to avoid drug interactions in the elderly.
- Abrupt withdrawal of clozapine may precipitate a withdrawal psychosis which is very difficult to treat.
- Clozapine may be an effective treatment for tardive dyskinesia.

References

Alvir JMM, Lieberman JA, Safferman AZ et al (1993) Clozapine induced agranulocytosis, *N Eng J Med* **329:** 162–7.

Chengappa KNR, Baker RW, Kreinbrook SB et al (1995) Clozapine use in female geriatric patients with psychosis, *J Geriatr Psychiatry Neurol* **8:** 12–15.

Cobb CD, Anderson CB, Scidel DR (1991) Possible interaction between clozapine and lorazepam, *Am J Psychiatry* **148:** 1606–7.

Ekblom B, Eriksson K, Lindstrom LH (1984) Supersensitivity psychosis in schizophrenic patients after sudden clozapine withdrawal, *Psychopharmacology* **83:** 293–4.

Frankenburg FR, Kalunion D (1994) Clozapine in the elderly, *J Geriatr Psychiatry Neurol* **7:** 131–4.

Grohmann R, Rüther E, Sassim N et al (1989) Adverse effects of clozapine, *Psychopharmacology* **99:** 5101–4.

Herst L, Powell G (1997) Is clozapine safe in the elderly? *Aust NZ J Psychiatry* **31:** 411–17.

Lieberman JA, Kane JM, Johns CA (1989) Clozapine: guidelines for clinical management, *J Clin Psychiatry* **50:** 329–38.

Lieberman JA, Saltz BL, Johns CA et al (1991) The effects of clozapine on tardive dyskinesia, *Br J Psychiatry* **158:** 503–10.

Meltzer HY, Ranjan R, Lee MA et al (1995) Emerging clinical uses of clozapine, *Rev Contemp Pharmacother* **6:** 187–96.

Palia SS, Clarke CJ (1993) Clozaril withdrawal syndrome, *Psychiatr Bull* **17:** 374–5.

Parsa MA, Al-Lahram YH, Ramirez LF et al (1993) Prolonged psychotic relapse after abrupt clozapine withdrawal, *J Clin Psychopharmacol* **13:** 154–5.

Ratey JJ, Leveroni C, Kilmer D et al (1993) The effects of clozapine on severely aggressive psychiatric inpatients in a State hospital, *J Clin Psychiatry* **54:** 219–23.

Sajatovic M, Jaskiw G, Konicki EP et al (1997) Outcome of clozapine therapy for elderly patients with refractory primary psychosis, *Int J Geriatr Psychiatry* **12:** 553–8.

Schulk JR (1985) Homicide and suicide associated with akathisia and haloperidol, *Am J Forensic Psychiatry* **6:** 3–7.

Taylor D (1997a) Switching from typical to atypical antipsychotics – practical guidelines, *CNS Drugs* **8:** 285–12.

Taylor D (1997b) Pharmacokinetic interactions involving clozapine, *Br J Psychiatry* **171:** 109–12.

Thompson C (1994) Consensus Statement: The use of high dose antipsychotic medication, *Br J Psychiatry* **164:** 448–58.

Negative symptoms

Carol Paton

PF, a 21-year-old man, was visited in a mental health aftercare hostel in order to administer his depot injection (fluphenazine decanoate 100 mg every two weeks). His keyworker reported increasing problems with PF's self care and motivation. It was increasingly difficult to persuade him to have a bath and he had not attended the day centre for several weeks. PF isolated himself in his room where he spent most of his time smoking in bed. The floor was covered in cigarette burns and staff were concerned about possible fire risk.

PF had been admitted to hospital briefly, aged 17, when he described derealisation and depersonalisation and some passivity phenomena. PF was known to be mis-using cannabis heavily at this time and a diagnosis of drug-induced psychosis was made. He received haloperidol 20 mg bd for three weeks in hospital, but discharged himself against medical advice and never attended out-

patients or his GP for further supplies. PF was again admitted, aged 20 'in a much deteriorated state' suffering from third person auditory hallucinations, thought disorder, and delusions about electrical equipment. These symptoms responded well to fluphenazine decanoate 100 mg every 2 weeks, but significant problems with self care, motivation and social skills remained.

PF is the only child of a single mother, was a forceps delivery and was slow to achieve milestones (walking age two, talking age two and a half). Physical examination noted an underweight young man with a squint in his left eye. He had marked psychomotor slowing, lack of facial expression and a resting tremor. Routine blood tests were normal. Urine drug screen was negative.

Questions

1. Which pharmacological interventions would be appropriate at this time?
2. Are traditional antipsychotics effective against primary negative symptoms?
3. Are atypical antipsychotics effective against primary negative symptoms?
4. Can any efficacy against primary negative symptoms in the acute phase of illness be generalised to patients with enduring negative symptoms?

Answers

1 Which pharmacological interventions would be appropriate at this time?

This patient's positive symptoms have responded well to fluphenazine depot and negative symptoms currently dominate the clinical picture. Negative symptoms of schizophrenia include alogia (poverty of speech/content), flattened/blunted affect, anhedonia, asociality, avolition/apathy and motor retardation. Subjective sadness, pessimism and suicidal intent are not considered to be negative symptoms (Coffey, 1994). Negative symptoms are generally considered to be more 'biological' in nature than positive symptoms and there are both organic and dynamic hypotheses. Negative symptoms have been associated with enlarged cerebral ventricles, intellectual impairment, lack of response to antipsychotics and poor prognosis

(Crow, 1980), and have been said to predict poor functioning in both the short and the long term (Pogue-Geile and Harrow, 1985). A biological aetiology for enduring negative symptoms (deficit state) is supported by EEG changes which are consistent with a 'hypofrontality' hypothesis. More severe negative symptoms and an earlier age of onset are associated with low interleukin-2 production which may reflect an autoimmune disturbance (reviewed by McPhillips & Barnes, 1997).

Negative symptoms may have many origins and it is important to determine the most likely cause in any individual case before embarking on a treatment regimen. This area is described in detail by Carpenter (1996), who describes negative symptoms as being either primary (transient or enduring), or secondary to positive symptoms (eg asociality secondary to paranoia), bradykinesia (EPSEs: lack of emotional spontaneity, retarded speech, few gestures, decreased movements), depression (eg anhedonia, social withdrawal, apathy) or institutionalisation. Primary transient negative symptoms must be differentiated from both primary enduring negative symptoms (deficit state) and secondary negative symptoms caused by anti-

psychotic side-effects. This is not a simple task, as these symptoms are not mutually exclusive and commonly co-exist.

The patient in this case has made a good response to fluphenazine with respect to positive symptoms. The negative symptoms that remain may be primary enduring negative symptoms or secondary to EPSEs or depression. The dose of depot prescribed is high and a reasonable first step would be to reduce this. Antipsychotic dosage reduction studies which have observed patients on long-term treatment through periods of dosage reduction have noted improvements in blunted affect, emotional withdrawal and psychomotor retardation (Marder et al, 1984). A trial of an anticholinergic, with the aim of reducing EPSEs, may also be worthwhile, as may a trial of an atypical antipsychotic (see question 3). Depending on further evaluation of the mental state, treatment with an antidepressant may be appropriate.

2. Are traditional antipsychotics effective against primary negative symptoms?

Clinical trials which demonstrate the efficacy of the older typical antipsychotics routinely show a 'broad spectrum' effect against both positive and negative symptoms in the acute phase. Negative symptoms are less likely to respond in the maintenance phase when positive symptoms are in remission. Early studies found that indifference to the environment, apathy, inappropriate affect, poor social participation and poor self care responded to antipsychotic treatment whereas these symptoms developed over time in placebo-treated patients (Goldberg et al, 1965). Waddington et al (1995) found that in a cohort of older patients with schizophrenia, an increased period of initial untreated psychosis led to an increased incidence later of poverty of speech. The earlier the antipsychotic treatment was started in this group, the less the decline over time.

These findings would be consistent with the hypotheses that:

• Primary negative symptoms may be secondary to positive symptoms where social withdrawal may be secondary to acute paranoid delusions (Carpenter, 1996).
• The earlier treatment with antipsychotics is started, the better the long-term outcome (Wyatt, 1995). Early effective treatment with antipsychotics has been shown to

alter the trajectory of decline and may prevent the development of enduring negative symptoms.

In conclusion, while conventional antipsychotics may treat negative symptoms that are secondary to acute positive symptoms, or decrease relapse rates and prevent the development of chronic symptoms, there is no evidence to show that they have significant efficacy against primary enduring negative symptoms. This is complicated by the observation that conventional antipsychotics may cause so-called secondary negative symptoms (due to EPSE).

3. Are atypical antipsychotics effective against primary negative symptoms?

Atypical antipsychotics are so named because they have at least equivalent antipsychotic potency to the older compounds but with significantly less potential for producing EPSEs. This may be due to their relative selectivity for mesolimbic dopamine pathways or their high 5HT2 : D2 blocking ratio or both. In clinical practice, most atypicals also show slightly superior efficacy to typicals in the treatment of positive symptoms and this may translate into improved social integration. Clozapine is uniquely effective in treatment-resistant illness. The atypicals risperidone, sertindole, olanzapine, quetiapine and clozapine might therefore be expected to treat positive symptoms perhaps without producing secondary negative symptoms. Whether atypicals have efficacy against negative symptoms beyond the secondary improvements from reduced positive symptoms and the relative lack of EPSEs is a moot point.

It has been postulated that serotonergic antagonism would counteract negative symptoms that may arise from hypodopaminergic pathophysiology in prefrontal cortical areas. Initial hope that potent 5HT2 blockade might be beneficial in the treatment of negative symptoms came from a study by Duinkerke et al (1993), in which ritanserin, a selective 5HT2 and 5HT1C antagonist, was added to stable treatment regimes with typical antipsychotics. Facial expression, flattened affect and relationships with friends and peers were all noted to improve.

Sertindole is an atypical antipsychotic which may be relatively selective for mesolimbic D2 pathways, has a high 5HT2 : D2 blocking ratio and has an incidence of EPSEs indistinguishable from that of placebo. In an efficacy trial (patients were not specifically selected for the presence of negative symptoms) which randomised 497 patients to receive sertindole 12, 20 or 24 mg, haloperidol 8 or 16 mg, or placebo for eight weeks, EPSEs occurred no more frequently with sertindole than with placebo. Using the Scale for the Assessment of Negative Symptoms (SANS; Andreasen, 1983), no dose of sertindole was more effective than any dose of haloperidol and only sertindole 20 mg was significantly more effective than placebo for negative symptoms (Zimbroff et al, 1997).

A meta-analysis of risperidone studies (Carman et al, 1995), which used the Positive and Negative Syndrome Scale (PANSS, Kay et al, 1987) and SANS scores to determine the severity of negative symptoms before and after risperidone treatment, concluded that patients were 1.5 times more likely to experience clinically significant reductions in negative symptoms with risperidone than with placebo. Risperidone was said to have an equal effect directly on primary negative symptoms, and indirectly through decreasing positive symptoms and EPSE or depression. However, by far the largest study included in this meta-analysis was that of Peuskens et al

(1995), where 450 patients received 4 or 8 mg risperidone and 222 patients received 10 mg haloperidol for eight weeks. There was no difference between treatment groups in the response of primary negative symptoms in this trial (p = 0.39). The results of the meta-analysis were probably influenced by the publication bias that operates in favour of positive findings when small patient numbers are included in trials.

In a trial of olanzapine efficacy, 335 patients (90% of whom had a chronic course with an acute exacerbation) were randomised to receive a low (mean 5 mg), medium (mean 10 mg) or high (mean 15 mg) dose of olanzapine, haloperidol or placebo (Tollefson et al, 1997). One hundred and thirty-nine patients completed the six-week trial and the data were analysed by 'intent to treat' analysis. The later the age at onset of illness, the greater the response of negative symptoms in this cohort. There was a positive relationship between improvements in negative symptoms and improvements in mood and EPSEs.

There are no published data for quetiapine demonstrating efficacy against negative symptoms superior to that shown by traditional antipsychotics. Indeed, most trials show equal efficacy.

Clozapine is uniquely effective in patients with treatment-resistant schizophrenia and the large study by Kane et al (1988) demonstrated superior efficacy to chlorpromazine for both positive and negative symptoms. The improvement in negative symptoms in this study could be explained by the very significant response of positive symptoms and lack of EPSEs.

4. Can any efficacy against primary negative symptoms in the acute phase of illness be generalised to patients with enduring negative symptoms?
Patients who have two or more moderately severe primary negative symptoms that are stable over the course of at least one year are said to have trait negative symptoms or the deficit state.

Amisulpride is an unconventional antipsychotic which has high affinity for D2 and D3 receptors. At low doses it blocks the presynaptic D3 autoreceptor, thus facilitating dopamine transmission, while at higher doses it blocks postsynaptic D2 receptors in the same manner as conventional antipsychotics. In a double blind, placebo-controlled trial of 104 patients (who had negative symptoms for a mean of eight years) randomised to receive amisulpride 100 mg, 300 mg or placebo for six weeks (Boyer et al, 1995), there was no change in positive symptoms or EPSEs across the three treatment groups, while both doses of active drug were significantly more effective than placebo against negative symptoms using ratings on SANS. Significant improvements in affective blunting, alogia, avolition/apathy and attentional impairment were seen in up to 50% of the amisulpride-treated patients compared with up to 25% of the placebo-treated patients. There was a pretreatment wash-out phase of six weeks to exclude improvements in secondary negative symptoms. These results are supported by a further randomised double-blind placebo-controlled trial in which 141 patients were treated with amisulpride 100 mg or placebo for six weeks (Loo et al, 1997). Patients were selected on the grounds of having a chronic illness with residual negative symptoms. Improvement was defined as a 50% reduction in baseline SANS score. Forty-two per cent of amisulpride patients improved compared with 15.5% of placebo patients. Again, significant improvements were seen in affective flattening, alogia, avolition/

apathy, anhedonia/asociality and attentional impairment, and these were not correlated with improvements in positive symptoms or EPSEs.

Amisulpride has been compared with low-dose haloperidol in 60 patients with predominant enduring negative symptoms in a randomised double-blind trial (Speller et al, 1997). This study followed patients over a period of one year while attempts at dosage reduction were made. The majority of patients randomised to amisulpride received a dose of 150 mg per day or less at the end of the trial period, while the majority of the haloperidol group received 4.5 mg per day or less. The effect of either treatment on negative symptoms was modest and, although the amisulpride group fared slightly better, the difference did not reach statistical significance.

In a 12-month open-label trial of 50 treatment-resistant patients, clozapine was found to have significant antipsychotic effect in both deficit and non-deficit patients (Conley et al, 1994). Improvement in negative symptoms was observed only in the non-deficit group. In a further double-blind efficacy trial of clozapine (Brier et al, 1994) in which 39 stable outpatients who were partial responders to previous antipsychotic regimens were randomised to receive 200–600 mg clozapine or 10–30 mg haloperidol daily for 10 weeks, clozapine was found to be significantly more effective than haloperidol in the treatment of both positive and negative symptoms. On further analysis, the significant difference in efficacy against negative symptoms was due to a modest decrease in the clozapine group combined with a modest increase in the haloperidol group. In the subgroup of patients in this trial who fulfilled the criteria for the deficit syndrome (n = 11), clozapine and haloperidol were equally effective against negative symptoms.

In conclusion, with the exception of low-dose amisulpride, which has shown a modest effect, no other typical or atypical antipsychotic has shown any significant efficacy against primary enduring negative symptoms. Further studies of other atypical antipsychotics are awaited.

Key points

- Negative symptoms can be primary (transient or enduring) or secondary to positive symptoms, depression, EPSEs or institutionalisation. Intervention is dependent upon aetiology.
- The earlier antipsychotic treatment is started, the less likely the patient is subsequently to develop negative symptoms.
- Traditional antipsychotics have limited efficacy against negative symptoms and can cause secondary negative symptoms (through their propensity to cause EPSEs).
- Atypical antipsychotics are less likely to cause EPSEs and, therefore, secondary negative symptoms than the older drugs, but are not convincingly more effective against primary negative symptoms.
- Clozapine is uniquely effective against resistant positive symptoms and is virtually devoid of EPSEs, properties which translate clinically into a very low incidence of secondary negative symptoms. It is not convincingly effective against primary enduring negative symptoms ('deficit state').
- Amisulpride in doses of 300 mg per day or less is the only antipsychotic with proven efficacy against primary enduring negative symptoms. This effect is modest.

References

Andreasen NC (1983) *The Scale for the Assessment of Negative Symptoms (SANS).* (Iowa City, IA: University of Iowa).

Boyer P, Lecrubier Y, Peuch AJ et al (1995) Treatment of negative symptoms in schizophrenia with amisulpride, *Br J Psychiatry* **166:** 68–72.

Breier A, Buchanan RW, Kirkpatrick B et al (1994) Effects of clozapine on positive and negative symptoms in outpatients with schizophrenia, *Am J Psychiatry* **151:** 20–6.

Carman J, Peuskens J, Vangeneugden A (1995) Risperidone in the treatment of negative symptoms of schizophrenia: a meta-analysis, *Int Clin Psychopharmacol* **10:** 207–13.

Carpenter WT (1996) The treatment of negative symptoms: pharmacological and methodological issues, *Br J Psychiatry* **168:**(suppl 29), 17–22.

Coffey I (1994) Negative symptoms of schizophrenia, *CNS Drugs* **1:**(2), 107–18.

Conley R, Gounaris C, Tamminga C (1994) Clozapine response varies in deficit versus non-deficit schizophrenic subjects, *Biol Psychiatry* **35:** 746–7.

Crow TJ (1980) Molecular pathology of schizophrenia; more than one disease process, *Br Med J* **11:** 471–86.

Duinkerke SJ, Botter PA, Jansen AA (1993) Ritanserin, a selective 5HT2/1C antagonist, and negative symptoms in schizophrenia, *Br J Psychiatry* **164:** 451–5.

Goldberg SC, Klerman GL, Cole JD (1965) Changes in schizophrenic psychopathology and ward behaviour as a function of phenothiazine treatment, *Br J Psychiatry* **111:** 120–33.

Kane J, Honigfeld G, Singer J et al (1988) Clozapine for the treatment resistant schizophrenic: a double blind comparison with chlorpromazine, *Arch Gen Psychiatry* **45:** 789–96.

Kay SR, Fiszbein A, Opler LA (1987) Positive and negative syndrome scale (PANSS) for schizophrenia, *Schizophrenia Bull* **13:** 261–76.

Loo H, Poirier-Littre MF, Theron M et al (1997) Amisulpride versus placebo in the medium term treatment of the negative symptoms of schizophrenia, *Br J Psychiatry* **170:** 18–22.

Marder SR, Van Putten T, Mintz J et al (1984) Costs and benefits of two doses of fluphenazine, *Arch Gen Psychiatry* **41:** 1025–9.

McPhillips MA, Barnes TRE (1997) Negative symptoms, *Curr Opin Psychiatry* **10:** 30–5.

Peuskens J and the Risperidone Study Group (1995) Risperidone in the treatment of chronic schizophrenic patients; a multi-national, multi-centre, double-blind, parallel group study versus haloperidol, *Br J Psychiatry* **166:** 712–26.

Pogue-Geile MF, Harrow M (1985) Negative symptoms in schizophrenia: their longitudinal course and prognostic importance, *Schizophrenia Bull* **85:** 11–12.

Speller JC, Barnes TRE, Curson DA et al (1997) One-year, low dose neuroleptic study of inpatients with chronic schizophrenia characterised by persistent negative symptoms, *Br J Psychiatry* **171:** 564–8.

Tollefson GD, Sanger TM (1997) Negative symptoms: a path analytical approach to a double blind, placebo and haloperidol controlled clinical trial with olanzapine, *Am J Psychiatry* **154:** 466–74.

Waddington JL, Youssef HA, Kinsella A (1995) Sequentional cross sectional and ten-year prospective study of severe negative symptoms in relation to duration of initially untreated psychosis in chronic schizophrenia, *Psychol Med* **25:** 849–57.

Wyatt RJ (1995) Early intervention for schizophrenia: can the course of the illness be altered? *Biol Psychiatry* **38:** 1–3.

Zimbroff DL, Kane JM, Tamminga CA (1997) Controlled, dose response study of sertindole and haloperidol in the treatment of schizophrenia, *Am J Psychiatry* **154:** 782–91.

Drug-induced psychosis

Railton Scott

5

SS, a 20-year-old Caucasian woman, was admitted
to the acute psychiatric unit after assessment in
casualty. She had been brought to hospital by
flatmates who were becoming increasingly
concerned by her 'bizarre' behaviour. Her friends
described two days of chaotic behaviour. SS had
hardly slept and had eaten very little. On direct
questioning her flatmates stated that SS was a
regular (most days) user of cannabis and 'might
also have taken amphetamines recently'. SS had
no psychiatric history and no known medical
problems.

On examination SS was very agitated, unable to
sit still and could not answer any questions in a
coherent way. She refused to believe that she was
in hospital but believed she had been taken to a
special police unit for 'super-humans'. These 'super-
humans' used drugs to attain higher states and
she stated that she would be held until she
revealed the names of her 'dealers and followers'.

SS continually uttered the phrase 'weed and speed, speed and weed'. She would not agree to physical examination but was noted to be sweating, and her pupils were dilated. Her respiratory rate was rapid.

SS, after much persuasion, accepted 10 mg of diazepam syrup. She settled within an hour and reluctantly allowed a blood and urine sample to be taken. She then accepted approximately 500 ml of orange juice and slept in her allocated side-room for over 12 hours.

Results urgently requested from biochemistry revealed a normal FBC,

U&Es, TFTs, LFTs, and random glucose. SS tested positive for cannabis and amphetamines. The working diagnosis was that of an acute drug-induced psychosis.

SS was treated with reducing doses of diazepam and her agitation continued to settle. Initial paranoid ideation and delusions of grandeur also resolved without use of antipsychotics, but she continued to complain of depersonalisation and derealisation for several weeks. Subsequent urine testing for drugs was clear, except for cannabis and her prescribed medication. She vehemently denied any subsequent drug misuse.

Questions

1. Describe common presenting features in a person suffering from the acute toxic effects of amphetamines and cannabis. How should these symptoms be treated in the case of SS?
2. Sequential urine testing gave the following results:
   Week 3: Cannabis +.
   Week 4: Cannabis ++.
   SS denied any further use of cannabis. Can these results be explained?
3. SS was discharged within two weeks of admission. What factors may influence SS with regard to future drug misuse? What, if any, on-going drug treatment is appropriate?
4. Which other drugs can induce psychotic symptoms?

Answers

1. Describe common presenting features in a person suffering from the acute toxic effects of amphetamines and cannabis. How should these symptoms be treated in the case of SS?

The acute effects of amphetamines ('speed', 'whizz', 'Billy', 'Berwick', etc) may be divided into central, cardio-vascular and gastrointestinal. Central effects include restlessness with hyper-reflexia, tremor, dizziness, excessive talking and possibly euphoria. If amphet-amine use had been sustained (a 'binge' or 'run') the presenting mood is more likely to be one of irritation and/or suspicion. Insomnia is common as are confusion and feelings of panic. Cardiovascular effects include headache, cardiac arrhyth-mias and anginal pain. Blood pressure is often labile with hyper- and hypotension both commonly occurring. Sweating and piloerection can occur ('clucking'). Gastrointestinal effects include anorexia, dry mouth and abdominal cramping with or without diarrhoea. Nausea and vomit-ing may occur (Weiner, 1980).

The acute effects of cannabis ('grass', 'weed', 'ganja', 'Mary-Jane', 'hash', etc) can be split into cardiovascular and central. Common cardiovascular effects include increases in heart rate and a drop in systolic blood pressure. Interestingly, there is often a marked reddening of the conjunctiva. Central effects are varied and range from mild euphoria to frank hallucinations, delusions and paranoid ideation. At relatively low doses there may be subjectively pleasant distortions of various auditory and visual stimuli.

Toxic effects may also include those caused directly by the user's chosen method of administration: cannabis may be smoked in a 'joint' or 'reefer' or may be eaten in the form of a 'hash' cake; occasionally marijuana may be made into an infusion ('bhang') and drunk. Toxic effects occur as a result of smoking and commonly include cough, wheeze and a dry throat (Nahas, 1977).

It should also be noted that cannabis will vary in its potency as a psychomimetic agent according to the proportion of the active ingredient – delta-9-tetrahydrocannabinoid (THC). Infusions may contain 1–10% THC as may the marijuana 'reefer', whilst the hashish resin may contain 8–15% THC. Hashish oil, extracted from the resin, may have a THC content as high as 60%. Isbell et al in 1967 were able to demonstrate that the psychomimetic effects of cannabis were dose dependent and that changes in mood (mostly euphoria) progressed to depersonalisation and derealisation with visual and auditory hallucinations on administration of higher doses of THC. Evidence that cannabis may cause an acute toxic psychosis comes mainly from countries such as the United States and Sweden. It is suspected that a lack of awareness and experience amongst doctors in the UK is resulting in an underdiagnosis of this condition (Poole and Brabbins, 1996). In addition, some researchers have argued for the existence of a chronic psychosis induced by cannabis (Negrete 1973, Chopra and Smith, 1974). Others have argued that because the drug has such a long half-life this represents chronic intoxication and not chronic psychosis.

It has long been accepted that the use of amphetamines can mimic symptoms of schizophrenia, especially if the individual is acutely intoxicated and is presenting with paranoia/paranoid ideation (Bell, 1973). Furthermore, experimentation involving amphetamines (specifically the acute toxic effects) has been used to develop the dopamine hypothesis of schizophrenia (Snyder et al, 1974).

From the history given – the admission of drug taking by SS – confirmed by the results of urine screening, it is accepted that SS has misused both cannabis and amphetamines. It is now essential to establish whether SS is presenting with 'pure' drug-induced psychosis or whether there is an underlying psychosis that requires treatment.

Thus there is now a diagnostic dilemma with SS. The differential diagnosis is between psychosis induced by amphetamine and/or cannabis, an independent psychotic illness or a combination of the two. Confirmation of the diagnosis may be established if the psychotic features persist beyond a specific time period and there has been no further substance misuse. This period is given as one month in DSM-IV. However, adopting this time frame may be both simplistic and misleading. Firstly, the spontaneous recurrence of hallucinations following amphetamine use has been widely reported (Keeler et al, 1968). Secondly, research has shown that following exposure to amphetamines some subjects are more sensitive to both repeated amphetamine exposure and, most significantly, other non-pharmacological stresses – e.g. shock, pain, fear, etc (Antelman, 1980).

Diagnosis also determines treatment strategy. Amphetamine-induced psychosis is best treated initially by benzodiazepines, for example, diazepam 10 mg orally or IV (Linden et al, 1985). If the patient fails to settle, a high potency antipsychotic such as haloperidol should be used (Angrist et al, 1974). Five milligrams orally or IM would be a suitable dose. Low potency phenothiazines are probably best avoided, owing to their ability to induce hypotension and tachycardia. In addition, the potent anticholinergic effects of these drugs may complicate management if other anticholinergic drugs of abuse have also been consumed. Low potency phenothiazines such as chlorpromazine are very sedative and this may contribute to the increased risk of respiratory depression when these agents are used to treat drug-induced psychoses (Dubin et al, 1986).

There are no data concerning the use of the new antipsychotics in drug-induced psychosis, although there is no reason to believe that they would not be as effective as the older drugs. It should be noted that risperidone, sertindole and quetiapine are all potent adrenergic alpha$_1$ blockers and olanzapine has significant anticholinergic effects. These properties, when shown by chlorpromazine, are thought to be undesirable, as discussed above.

2. Sequential urine testing gave the following results:

Week 3: Cannabis +.

Week 4: Cannabis ++.

SS denied any further use of cannabis. Can these results be explained?

When cannabis is smoked, peak plasma levels of THC occur within 10–30 minutes. THC is very lipophilic, leaving the blood stream rapidly and being stored in body adipose tissue, from which it is slowly released back into the blood stream. The elimination half-life is approximately 7–8 days. If cannabis use is repeated at intervals of less than the half-life of THC then accumulation of THC and its metabolites will occur. The detection of THC by urine analysis will depend on factors such as the assay method used and whether use had been acute or chronic. Acute use can be detected by urine analysis for at least a week following the administration of cannabis. Chronic use may result in detection after four weeks or longer (Garrett, 1979). Passive smoking may also result in a positive urine test for cannabis (Zeidenberg et al, 1977).

The picture is further complicated by the observation that the urine drug concentration may change by a factor of 10 in a matter of hours. As THC has a long half-life, detection is probable over several weeks. Also, if there was a high fluid intake and the drug concentration was approaching the 'cut-off' level of the assay used, then this may result in a reduced positive (+) or even negative reading. Subsequent restricted fluid intake would concentrate the urine which could result in a *relative* increase in THC concentration and a result of (++) (Simpson et al, 1997).

3. SS was discharged with two weeks of admission. What factors may influence SS with regard to future drug misuse? What, if any, on-going drug treatment is appropriate?

SS has misused both amphetamines and cannabis. Amphetamine is a drug with strong and immediate reinforcing properties and so the potential for relapse is high (Schuckit, 1994). The nature and extent of the withdrawal syndrome may also influence whether SS will return to drug misuse (Lago and Kosten, 1994). Although the acute phase of withdrawal has been reported to peak at 2–4 days, symptoms may persist for several weeks (Gessop et al, 1982).

Once the patient is away from the supportive influence of the hospital environment with the added security of inpatient status, the temptation to 'use' again may be strong. SS may benefit from various strategies aimed at rehabilitation. This has been described as a three-step process (Schuckit, 1994). A detailed analysis is beyond the scope of this book, so the following is a brief summary. The first step involves education of both users and their family/friends. The second step uses counselling – both group and individual. Attendance at a self-help group is also encouraged. The third and final step is aimed at relapse prevention. Situations and moods when craving is likely to be most intense are identified and strategies to deal with the cravings are then devised.

In summary, rehabilitation of substance misusers involves behavioural, cognitive and psychological processes. It begins during detoxification but is most intense after acute withdrawal. Patients are then encouraged to attend counselling and self-help groups, for many months is some cases, following the initial intense stage.

Appropriate detoxification and re-habilitation programmes result in a maximum improvement rate of 20–40% as measured by continued abstinence and fewer life problems in the subsequent year (Meyer, 1992). Overall the response rate is relatively modest. In an attempt to boost this, the role of pharmacological interventions is continually being investigated. It should be noted, however, that proving efficacy for any drug treatment in the field of substance dependence is difficult. The intensity of craving fluctuates, and there is a considerable rate of spontaneous remission (Schuckit, 1994). There are few treatments that have been properly validated in large treatment groups by adopting the classical double-blind controlled procedure with a placebo or standard therapy as control (Meyer, 1992).

Amphetamines influence at least three neurochemical systems: dopamine (DA), noradrenaline (NA) and serotonin (5-HT). It has been postulated that chronic stimulant misuse results in decreased functioning of the dopamine pathways (Kranzler and Bauer, 1992). For this reason bromocriptine, a dopamine agonist, was extensively investigated, but after promising early results more recent and better controlled trials have not supported its usefulness (Kransler and Bauer, 1992). Other trials with DA-boosting drugs such as mazindol

(Teronac) and amantadine have also been disappointing (Tennant and Sagherian, 1987).

Two other neurotransmitter systems open to modification are those involving noradrenaline and serotonin. Treatment choice centres on appropriate antidepressant medication, designed to boost NA and 5-HT levels. Positive results were achieved by using the tricyclic antidepressant desipramine (now discontinued) in an early trial (Kosten et al, 1987), but this was an open, uncontrolled trial and subsequent work with a larger sample failed to demonstrate any superiority of desipramine over placebo (Kosten et al, 1992).

More recent work has investigated the use of anticonvulsants such as carbamazepine, which is thought to act by reducing the kindling effect of stimulants, and antidepressants such as fluoxetine, which act more specifically on the 5-HT system (Halikas et al, 1992; Balki et al, 1993). Further trial work needs to be carried out with large patient numbers in well-controlled trials before evidence-based recommendations can be made.

Obviously, if any patient is suspected of co-morbidity such as social phobia, depression or bipolar affective disorder then this must be treated and would influence the specific agents used in the patient being treated for stimulant dependence.

In summary, SS has been detoxified from amphetamines and cannabis. She has made a good recovery but some symptoms remain. She should be closely followed up on discharge and the diagnosis and subsequent treatment should be reviewed as necessary. Dealing with drug-induced psychosis can be difficult, owing to the possibility of co-morbidity, and drug treatment must be prescribed with care. The effectiveness of such treatment should be closely monitored and evaluated, with alterations being made as the situation dictates.

4. Which other drugs can induce psychotic symptoms?

Many drugs, both illicit and prescribed, have been linked to the emergence of psychotic symptoms. Many mechanisms may be involved including the induction of delirium or intoxication, the precipitation or worsening of existing psychoses and withdrawal psychoses. Drugs of abuse include cannabis, amphetamines, diamorphine, cocaine, ecstasy, khat, LSD, phencyclidine, solvents,

ephedrine and alcohol. The withdrawal of benzodiazepines, nicotine, clozapine and anticholinergics has also been implicated, as have the prescription drugs vigabatrin, selegiline, propranolol, enalapril, chloroquine, steroids, cimetidine and sulphonamides. For a comprehensive, well-referenced list, see Bazire (1997).

Key points

- Drug-induced psychosis should initially be treated by a benzodiazepine. If response is inadequate, a modest dose of antipsychotic should be prescribed.
- Drug-induced psychosis is defined as lasting not more than one month following ingestion of the responsible substance.
- Co-morbidity is common and differential diagnosis can be difficult.
- Cannabis can be detected in the urine for four weeks or longer after the last administration in chronic use. A positive urine test does not confirm acute intoxication.
- Many drugs have been investigated for the prevention of relapse, but with little effect.
- Many drugs, both illicit and prescription, can induce psychotic symptoms.

References

Antelman SM (1980) Interchangeability of stress and amphetamines in sensitisation, *Science* **207**: 329–31.

Angrist B, Lee HK, Gershon S (1974) The antagonism of amphetamine-induced symptomatology by a neuroleptic, *Am J Psychiatry* **131**: 817–19.

Balki SL, Manfredi LB, Jacob P, Jones RT (1993) Fluoxetine for cocaine dependence in methadone maintenance, *J Clin Psychopharmacol* **13**: 243–50.

Bazire S (1997) Drug induced psychiatric disorders. In: *Psychotropic Drug Directory*, Quay Books. (Salisbury: Mark Allen Publishing) 233–52.

Bell DS (1973) The experimental reproduction of amphetamine psychosis, *Arch Gen Psychiatry* **29**: 35–40.

Chopra GS, Smith JW (1974) Psychotic reactions following cannabis use in East Indians, *Arch Gen Psychiatry* **30**: 24–7.

Dubin WR, Weiss KJ, Dorn JM (1986) Pharmacotherapy of psychiatric emergencies, *J Clin Psychopharmacol* **6**: 210–22.

Garrett ER (1979) Pharmacokinetics and disposition of delta (9) tetrahydrocannabinol and its metabolites. In: Nahas CG, Pahon W.M, eds. *Marijuana Biological Effects*. (Elmford, New York: Pergamon Press), 105–21.

Gessop MR, Bradley BP, Brewis RK (1982) Amphetamine withdrawal and sleep disturbance, *Drug Alcohol Depend* **10**: 177–83.

Halikas JA, Kuhn KL, Carlson G, Crea F, Crosby R (1992) The effect of carbamazepine on cocaine use, *Am J Addict* **1**: 30–9.

Isbell H, Gerodetzsky CW, Janiski D (1967) Effects of (–) delta-9-trans tetrahydrocannabinoid in man, *Psychopharmacologia* **11**: 184–8.

Keeler MH, Reifler CB, Liptzin MB (1968) Spontaneous recurrence of marijuana effect, *Am J Psychiatry* **125**: 364–8.

Kosten TR, Morgan CM, Falcione J, Schotlenfield RS (1992) Pharmacotherapy for cocaine-abusing methadone-maintained patients using amantidine or desipramine, *Arch Gen Psychiatry* **49**: 894–8.

Kosten TR, Schumann B, Wright D, Carney MK, Gavin FH (1987) A preliminary study of desipramine in the treatment of cocaine abuse, *J Clin Psychiatry* **48**: 442–4.

Kranzler HR, Bauer LO (1992) Bromocriptine and cocaine cue reactivity in cocaine dependent patients, *Br J Addict* **87**: 1537–48.

Lago JA, Kosten TR (1994) Stimulant withdrawal, *Addiction* **89:** 1477–81.

Linden CH, Kulig KW, Rumack BH (1985) Amphetamines. *Top Emerg Med* **7:** 18–32.

Meyer RE (1992) New pharmacotherapies for cocaine dependence revisited, *Arch Gen Psychiatry* **49:** 900–4.

Nahas G (1977) Biomedical aspects of cannabis usage, *Narc Bull* **24:** 13–27.

Negrete JC (1973) Psychological adverse effects of cannabis smoking – a tentative classification, *Can Med Assoc J* **108:** 195–202.

Poole R, Brabbins C (1996) Drug induced psychosis, *Br J Psychiatry* **168:** 135–8.

Schuckit MA (1994) The treatment of stimulant dependence, *Addiction* **89:** 1559–63.

Simpson D, Braithwaite RA, Janie DR, Stewart MJ (1997) Screening for drugs of abuse (ii); cannabinoids, lysergic acid diethylamide, buprenorphine, methadone, barbiturates, benzodiazepines and other drugs, *Ann Clin Biochem* **34:** 460–510.

Snyder SH, Banerjee SP, Yamamura HI, Greenberg D (1974) Drugs, neurotransmitters and schizophrenia, *Science* **184:** 1243–53.

Tennant FS, Sagherian AA (1987) Double blind comparison of amantidine and bromocriptine for ambulatory withdrawal from cocaine dependence, *Arch Intern Med* **147:** 109–12.

Weiner N (1980) Norepinephrine, epinephrine and the sympathomimetic agents. In: Gilman AG, Goodman LS, Gilman A, eds. *The Pharmacological Basis of Therapeutics.* (New York: Macmillan).

Zeidenberg P, Bourdon R, Nahas CG (1977) Marijuana intoxication by passive inhalation: documentation by detection of urinary metabolites, *Am J Psychiatry* **134:** 76–7.

Rapid tranquillisation

David Taylor

6

AH, a 38-year-old Caucasian man, was admitted to a locked, acute psychiatric care ward, having been brought in by the police. He was found praying by the side of the road, but became abusive and physically threatening when a policeman approached him. AH was reported to be 'making no sense at all – just talking incoherently about CNN' (the news' broadcaster).

On examination, AH was found to be severely thought-disordered, with fixed delusions about his role as head of CNN. He wore a hat at all times because it apparently protected him from the 'flat space invaders from CNN' by protecting his brain which 'is like the yolk inside the white, inside the brown'. AH became abusive before any more information could be gained. Having threatened nursing staff, he was restrained and secluded.

In seclusion, AH shouted that he wanted to kill himself and would 'take out anyone who got in his way'. It transpired that AH had no psychiatric history, but a long forensic record, including GBH, ABH and possession of an offensive weapon. He was taking no medication.

Questions

1. What are the aims of rapid tranquillisation?
2. What place do IM chlorpromazine and IM zuclopenthixol acetate have in AH's immediate treatment?
3. Outline a treatment plan for AH. List the safety measures necessary to ensure patient well-being.

Answers

1. What are the aims of rapid tranquillisation?

The principal aim of rapid tranquillisation (RT) is to reduce suffering and, in doing so, to do no harm to the patient. Thus it is no different from any other area of medicine. Secondary considerations include preventing self harm; preventing harm to others; and reducing the level of expressed emotion in the clinical environment.

RT is often used in psychiatric institutions for a variety of reasons. Acutely disturbed or violent behaviour can be a manifestation of many disorders, such as psychosis, substance abuse, stress reactions, dementia, organic disorders (eg cerebral tumours) and epilepsy. With such a range of possible precipitants, it is unlikely that any one medication or psychological approach would be suitable for all episodes of violent or disturbed behaviour. Thus, another central aim of RT is to ensure a flexible approach based on diagnosis and circumstance. In this case, the cause of the psychosis is unknown and a full physical and mental state examination, along with a comprehensive history, should be completed as soon as possible.

It should also be recognised that prevention of acutely disturbed or violent behaviour (usually by skilled nursing care and appropriate placement) is preferred to the essentially remedial RT. Where RT is required, as it will be even where preventative measures are in place, it is best managed and delivered by an expert or 'emergency' team of clinicians.

2. What place do IM chlorpromazine and IM zuclopenthixol acetate have in AH's immediate treatment?

Parenteral medication has no place in the immediate management of this patient. The use of parenteral antipsychotics, benzodiazepines and other sedatives should not be seen as first-line options in RT (Kerr and Taylor, 1997).

Initial management should involve the consideration of non-drug methods such as talking-down, distraction and, as in this case, seclusion. A full discussion of these methods is beyond the scope of this book. Nevertheless, it is important to recognise that non-drug methods are a humane, safe and often effective treatment for acutely disturbed behaviour.

Depending on diagnosis, oral medication may be appropriate and may be used alongside non-drug measures. With AH, psychosis is evident, although its cause is not known. Oral antipsychotic medication may thus be appro-priate and may engender sufficient improvement in the patient for a full history to be taken and for a mental state and physical examination to be completed. The main danger of using an antipsychotic with AH is that severe dystonia may occur: AH is apparently antipsychotic-naïve. Oral chlorpro-mazine (100 mg bd or tds) or haloperi-dol (2 mg bd) may be given (note these low, but therapeutic, doses). Droperidol has the advantage, should adverse effects be severe, of a short plasma half-life. An appropriate dose is 5 mg tds.

Newer, atypical drugs are probably effective in acute psychosis, although clinical experience is limited. The danger of dystonia is minimal, especially if low doses are used. However, the necessity for slow titra-tion with risperidone, sertindole and quetiapine arguably precludes their use in acute psychosis. Olanzapine 10 mg/day may be suitable and it has sedative properties which may be helpful. Ziprasidone seems to be effec-tive in acute psychosis and has anxio-lytic effects (Davis and Markham, 1997).

Intramuscular chlorpromazine remains a popular therapy in RT (Cunnane, 1994; Simpson and Anderson, 1996).

However, many now do not recommend its use (Kerr and Taylor, 1997). Absorption from IM administration is slow and erratic and varies substantially between individuals (Milton and Jann, 1995). Moreover, IM chlorpromazine can cause profound sedation and hypotension, especially in patients not previously exposed to neuroleptics. There also appears to be a tendency to use huge doses, very probably inappropriately (Mannion et al, 1997). Certainly IM chlorpromazine is unsuitable for this patient. Indeed, its use in any situation should be actively discouraged.

Zuclopenthixol acetate (Acuphase), a short-acting depot, is also widely used in RT despite a dearth of supporting literature (Coutinho et al, 1997). Because of the potential for prolonged dystonic reactions, this preparation is unsuitable for neuroleptic-naïve patients. It is also unsuitable for acute treatment. After injection, sedative effects are not apparent for at least two hours and peak at 24 hours (Chakravarti et al, 1990). Duration of action is two to three days (Amdisen et al, 1987). Zuclopenthixol acetate is best reserved for patients who otherwise need repeated injections of simple IM or IV formulations. In these situations it is claimed that fewer injections of zuclopenthixol acetate can be given to achieve the same effect as a large number of injections of shorter-acting preparations (Baastrup et al, 1993), although available data would suggest that the administration of additional antipsychotic medication is unlikely to be completely avoided (Fenton et al, 1997).

3. Outline a treatment plan for AH. List the safety measures necessary to ensure patient well-being.

Treatment plan

The following plan is recommended:

- First, try psychological methods, eg talking-down, time-out.
- Offer oral antipsychotic medication.
- If oral medication is refused, parenteral medication should be used if the patient remains severely distressed or is thought liable to cause harm to himself or others.

It is now common practice to give small doses of antipsychotics in combination with benzodiazepines. Intravenous administration is fast-acting and gives 100% bioavailability. It may, however, expose the heart to high concentrations of potentially cardiotoxic drugs. Intramuscular administration is slower-acting with less predictable absorption but is considered by some to be safer than the IV route.

Suggested regimens are:

> Haloperidol   5 mg IV
> +
> Diazepam   10 mg IV
>
> or
>
> Droperidol   10 mg IM
> +
> Lorazepam   1 mg IM

- Injections may be repeated if necessary after careful assessment – wait 15 minutes after IV injection; 30 minutes after IM injection.
- If the patient improves, offer oral medication.
- If the patient needs repeated injections, consider giving zuclopenthixol acetate (50–150 mg).
- In very extreme circumstances amylobarbitone 500 mg IM may be given. Full discussion with a consultant experienced in its use should ALWAYS precede administration.
- Instant access to ITU facilities should be available.

These recommendations are drawn from the recent review of Kerr and Taylor (1997).

Measures to ensure safety

- Parenteral procyclidine should be available in case of dystonic reaction.
- Flumazenil should be available to reverse the effects of benzodiazepines should respiratory depression occur. Staff should be familiar with its use.
- Monitoring should include:
  Pulse
  Temperature
  Blood pressure
  Respiratory rate
  Oxygen saturation (by pulse oximeter)
- Electrocardiograph (where available) (Note that training in ECG interpretation for psychiatric trainees is poor (Henderson et al, 1997), and advice should be sought if there is any doubt.)
- Full cardiac/resuscitation facilities should be available, preferably supplied by a 'crash team' in the same hospital.

Key points

- The principal aims of RT are to reduce suffering for the patient and make the environment safe for others.

- With skilled nursing management, only a small proportion of 'incidents' should result in RT.
- Oral medication should be offered first and may be sufficient.
- If the parenteral route is required, either haloperidol 5 mg and diazepam 10 mg IV or droperidol 10 mg and lorazepam 1 mg are recommended.
- Parenteral chlorpromazine is not recommended.
- Acuphase should never be given to antipsychotic-naïve patients because of its long duration of action, which will make difficult management of any acute dystonic reaction that may occur.
- Routine monitoring after RT should include TPR and BP. ECG monitoring is desirable.

References

Amdisen A, Nielsen MS, Dencker SJ et al (1987) Zuclopenthixol acetate in Viscoleo® in patients with acute psychoses including mania and exacerbation of chronic psychoses, *Acta Psychiatr Scand* **75:** 99–107.

Baastrup PC, Alhfors UG, Bjerkenstedt L et al (1993) A controlled Nordic multicentre study of zuclopenthixol acetate in oil solution, haloperidol and zuclopenthixol in the treatment of acute psychosis, *Acta Psychiatr Scand* **87:** 48–58.

Chakravarti SK, Muthu A, Muthu PK et al (1990) Zuclopenthixol acetate (5% in Viscoleo): single-dose treatment for acutely disturbed psychotic patients, *Curr Med Res Opin* **12:** 58–65.

Coutinho E, Fenton M, David A (1997) Details of studies of zuclopenthixol acetate are needed, *Br Med J* **315:** 884.

Cunnane JG (1994) Drug management of disturbed behaviour by psychiatrists, *Psychiatr Bull* **18:** 138–9.

Davis R, Markham A (1997) Ziprasidone, *CNS Drugs* **8:** 153–8.

Fenton M, Coutinho E, Campbell C (1997) Zuclopenthixol acetate in the treatment of acute schizophrenia and similar serious mental illness. In: Adams CE, Duggan L, de Jesus Mari J, White P, eds. Schizophrenia module of *The Cochrane Database of Systematic Reviews*. Available in the Cochrane Library. The Cochrane Collaboration, Issue 4, updated quarterly. (Oxford: Updated Software).

Henderson T, Gallagher D, Stark C (1997) A survey of the use of the electrocardiogram in psychiatry, *Psychiatr Bull* **21:** 136–8.

Kerr IB, Taylor D (1997) Acute disturbed or violent behaviour: principles of treatment, *J Psychopharmacol* **11:** 271–7.

Mannion L, Sloan D, Connolly L (1997) Rapid tranquillisation: are we getting it right? *Psychiatr Bull* **20:** 411–13.

Milton GV, Jann MW (1995) Emergency treatment of psychotic symptoms: pharmacokinetic considerations for antipsychotic drugs, *Clin Pharmacokinet* **28:** 494–504.

Simpson D, Anderson I (1996) Rapid tranquillisation: a questionnaire survey of practice, *Psychiatr Bull* **20:** 149–52.

Adherence to antipsychotic medication

Jennie Day

7

BT, a 46-year-old man who has had a diagnosis of schizophrenia for over 20 years, had again stopped taking both his depot and his oral antipsychotics. BT has had eight previous admissions to hospital and on four of these occasions he had stopped his medication within the previous six months. BT believes that in the past evil spirits had come upon him and made him speak in tongues, and that taking medication is irrelevant to these problems. He has been readmitted on previous occasions while taking medication, reinforcing his beliefs that it is irrelevant to his personal circumstances. BT has religious delusions which are only marginally attenuated by antipsychotics and at present he shows no signs of serious relapse.

Questions

1. What proportion of people with a diagnosis of schizophrenia do not adhere to medication regimens and how does this compare with other populations of medical patients?
2. How does non-adherence affect outcome in schizophrenia?
3. What factors may affect BT's decision to adhere to medication?
4. What strategies improve adherence to antipsychotics?

Answers

1. What proportion of people with a diagnosis of schizophrenia do not adhere to medication regimens and how does this compare with other populations of medical patients?

Around 50% of people with a diagnosis of schizophrenia do not adhere fully to medication regimens (Kane, 1985). Although this figure may seem high, in fact it is no higher than for other groups of people with chronic illnesses such as diabetes or hypertension (Ley, 1992).

2. How does non-adherence affect outcome in schizophrenia?

Non-adherence to antipsychotic medication is clinically significant. Discontinuing antipsychotics carries an increased risk of relapse (Kissling, 1994), and there is a well-established association between non-adherence to antipsychotics and rehospitalisation (Green, 1988). Non-adherence has been cited as the single most important cause of return of psychotic symptoms and readmission to hospital, and as a major preventable cause of psychiatric morbidity (Kane, 1983). However, it is important to stress that adherence is only appropriate if the drug is effective, lacking in distressing side-effects and tailored to the needs of the individual. Given the wide range of serious and distressing side-effects of antipsychotics and the relatively high rate of poor response, this raises problems. BT is probably a 'partial responder', in that he remains deluded when taking antipsychotics, but may cope slightly better with his delusions. This makes it difficult to argue from a therapeutic viewpoint that adherence is essential for continued well-being.

3. What factors may affect BT's decision to adhere to medication?

The reasons for taking or not taking medication are similar for psychiatric and non-psychiatric patients and are extremely complex. Perhaps unexpectedly side-effects of medication and psychological symptoms have only a minor role in affecting the decision to take antipsychotics. Health beliefs, subjective response to antipsychotics (including dysphoria) and personal attitudes to medication and psychiatry have a greater contribution (Kelly et al, 1987; Awad et al, 1996). A rating scale devised to measure attitudinal factors that influence adherence (Weiden et al, 1994) describes three subclasses related to adherence (influence of others; belief that medication would prevent relapse; feeling better on treatment) and five subscales related to non-adherence (dysphoria; problems obtaining medication; negative family influence; negative therapeutic alliance; rejection of an illness label). This scale is considered cumbersome by many workers, and some prefer the shorter Drug Attitude Inventory (Hogan and Awad, 1983).

Lack of insight has frequently been cited as an important contributor to non-adherence (e.g. Bartko et al, 1990), although the relationship between adherence and insight is more complex than it may at first appear. For example, some patients may continue taking medication even though they have little insight and other patients may have full insight but make an informed choice not to take medication. A number of insight scales include a negative attitude to medication as an indicator of lack of insight, but this overlooks the fact that people can make a logical and informed decision to discontinue medication independently of insight. In the case of BT it seems that lack of insight may be contributing to his decision not to take medication, as he may perceive side-effects and suboptimal response.

Another important predictor of adherence to medication regimens is the therapeutic alliance (Frank and Gunderson, 1990). Poor interpersonal skills of the prescriber, poor rapport between the patient and the prescriber and unresponsiveness to patients' complaints about side-effects have all been found to be related to lower rates of adherence.

4. What strategies improve adherence to antipsychotics?

There are many studies that have investigated interventions designed to improve adherence to antipsychotic treatment. Most of these studies have used an educational approach, assuming that if people have improved information about medication they are more likely to take it as prescribed. However, whilst this approach often leads to an improvement in knowledge about antipsychotics, it mostly does not lead to an improvement in adherence (Macpherson et al, 1996). Likewise, patients can be informed fully of the potential to develop tardive dyskinesia as a side-effect of antipsychotic drugs with little effect on their willingness to accept treatment (Chaplin and Kent, 1998). Behavioural approaches, where the medication is tailored to an individual's lifestyle, have been found to be more effective in increasing adherence (Boczkowski et al, 1985). More recently Kemp et al (1996) used a motivational interviewing-based intervention 'compliance therapy', which improved adherence, attitudes to treatment, insight and global functioning in people with a diagnosis of schizophrenia. Later work has shown that compliance therapy can prolong survival in community care (i.e. prevent re-admission) (Kemp et al, 1998). Thus in the case of BT an open and negotiating approach using such an intervention may be successful in improving his adherence. Atypical antipsychotics may be considered for BT, as there is some evidence that for risperidone, at least, some patients may feel subjectively better than when treated with the older drugs (Franz et al, 1997). Alternatively, since he has shown poor response to typical antipsychotics, the atypical antipsychotic clozapine could be tried in order to provide better symptomatic control. However, there is no good evidence that the atypical antipsychotics are associated with better rates of adherence, and moreover they are unlikely to change an individual's health beliefs.

Key points

- Approximately 50% of people with a diagnosis of schizophrenia do not adhere to their medication regimen. This proportion is similar to that found in other chronic illnesses such as diabetes or hypertension.
- Non-adherence increases relapse and re-hospitalisation.
- Perceived side-effects, health beliefs, subjective response to antipsychotics, perceived therapeutic alliance, influence of others, insight and the acceptance of an illness label all influence adherence to treatment.

- Education leads to improved knowledge, but has little impact on adherence.
- The motivational interviewing-based intervention, 'compliance therapy', has been shown to improve adherence, attitudes to treatment, insight, global functioning and survival in the community.

References

Awad AG, Voruganti LN, Heselgrave RJ et al (1996) Assessment of the patients' subjective experience in acute neuroleptic treatment: implications for compliance and outcome, *Int J Clin Psychopharmacol* **11:** 55–9.

Bartko G, Frecska E, Horvath S et al (1990) Predicting neuroleptic response from a combination of multilevel variables in acute schizophrenia patients, *Acta Psychiatr Scand* **82:** 408–12.

Boczkowski JA, Zeichner A, Desanto N (1985) Neuroleptic compliance among chronic schizophrenic outpatients, *J Consult Clin Psychol* **53:** 666–71.

Chaplin R, Kent A (1998) Informing patients about tardive dyskinesia: controlled trial of patient education, *Br J Psychiatry* **172:** 78–81.

Frank AF, Gunderson JG (1990) The role of therapeutic alliance in the treatment of schizophrenia, *Arch Gen Psychiatry* **47:** 228–36.

Franz M, Lis S, Pludderman K et al (1997) Conventional versus atypical neuroleptics: subjective quality of life in schizophrenic patients, *Br J Psychiatry* **170:** 422–5.

Green JH (1988) Frequent re-hospitalisation and non-compliance treatment, *Hosp Commun Psychiatry* **39:** 963–6.

Hogan TP, Awad AG and Eastwood MR (1983) A self-report scale predictive of drug compliance in schizophrenia, *Psych Med* **13:** 177–83.

Kane JM (1983) Problems of compliance in the outpatient treatment of schizophrenia, *J Clin Psychiatry* **44:** 3–6.

Kane JM (1985) Compliance issues in outpatient treatment, *J Clin Psychopharmacol* **5:** 22S–27S.

Kelly GR, Mamon JA, Scott JE (1987) Utility of the health belief model in examining medication compliance among psychiatric outpatients, *Soc Sci Med* **11:** 1205–11.

Kemp R, Hayward P, Applewhaile G et al (1996) Compliance therapy in psychotic patients: a randomised controlled trial, *Br Med J* **312:** 345–9.

Kemp R, Kirov G, Everitt B et al (1998) Randomised controlled trial of compliance therapy, *Br J Psych* **172:** 413–19.

Kissling W (1994) Compliance, quality assurance and standards for relapse prevention in schizophrenia, *Acta Psychiatr Scand* **89:** 16–24.

Ley P (1992) The problem of patients' non-compliance. In: *Communicating with Patients. Improving Communication, Satisfaction and Compliance.* (London: Chapman and Hall).

Macpherson R, Jerrom B, Hughes A (1996) A controlled study of education about drug treatment in schizophrenia, *Br J Psychiatry* **168:** 709–17.

Weiden P, Rapkin B, Mott T et al (1994) Rating of medication influences (ROMI) scale in schizophrenia, *Schizophr Bull* **20:** (2) 297–310.

Managing adverse effects of antipsychotics

Jennie Day

8

MB, a 23-year-old man, was admitted to an acute psychiatric ward via casualty. His mother had taken him to casualty because he had become increasingly paranoid and anxious and had tried to run across a very busy main road. MB presented with thought disorder and paranoid delusions, believing that MI5 were conspiring to kill him. He also had ideas of reference related to this and appeared agitated and anxious.

MB lived at home with a younger sister and his mother. His father had died 12 months before. MB's childhood appears to have been relatively normal; he achieved A levels and went on to work in a bank until he recently became ill. His mother reported that he had become increasingly withdrawn over the previous three months and in the last weeks before his admission had avoided social contact and work. There was no known history of any mental disorder in MB's family.

He was prescribed haloperidol 5 mg tds and procyclidine 5 mg tds and a urine drug screen was requested. The urine drug screen revealed no illicit drugs and a temporary working diagnosis of acute schizophrenia-like psychotic disorder was made. Unfortunately MB developed an oculogyric crisis. Haloperidol

was therefore discontinued and thioridazine 100 mg tds was prescribed.

Amongst other side-effects, MB became withdrawn on this medication and lacked motivation, which worried his family because they felt he would not return to work.

Questions

1. What chemical groups do haloperidol and thioridazine belong to, and, with reference to their pharmacological action, how do their side-effect profiles compare?
2. How is oculogyric crisis best managed?
3. What are the main measures used to assess the side-effects of antipsychotics and what are their strengths and weaknesses?
4. What syndrome could be responsible for the lack of motivation experienced by MB and how is it best managed?

Answers

1. What chemical groups do haloperidol and thioridazine belong to, and, with reference to their pharmacological action, how do their side-effect profiles compare?

Haloperidol is a butyrophenone and thioridazine is a piperidine phenothiazine. Butyrophenones are potent and fairly specific dopamine antagonists in the nigrostriatal pathway and this leads to increased extrapyramidal side-effects

(EPSEs) with this drug compared with most other antipsychotics. Thioridazine blocks muscarinic as well as dopamine receptors in the nigrostriatal pathway and this attenuates the disturbance of striatal function and thereby reduces the incidence of extrapyramidal side-effects. Unfortunately, whilst the central blockade of muscarinic receptors reduces the incidence of extrapyramidal side-effects, peripheral blockade leads to an increased incidence of side-effects such as dry mouth, blurred vision, constipation and urinary retention. Thioridazine is also a potent alpha$_1$-adrenergic antagonist, and this leads in particular to sexual problems which occur in approximately 60% of people prescribed thioridazine (Sullivan and Lukoff, 1990; Kotin et al, 1976). Alpha$_1$-adrenergic blockade also leads to a higher incidence of postural hypotension and nasal congestion. Thioridazine, like chlorpromazine, is a low potency phenothiazine and a dose of 300 mg/day is likely to be sedative, but perhaps unlikely to be antipsychotic. Thioridazine is best avoided in high antipsychotic doses over prolonged periods of time because of its ability to cause pigmentary retinopathy.

2. How is oculogyric crisis best managed?
Oculogyric crisis, an acute dystonic reaction, is a type of EPSE which usually occurs within the first five days of treatment. It is characterised by acute muscular spasm and results in an upward rotation of the eye which may leave the irises hidden behind the upper lids. This can be an extremely distressing side-effect and it is easy to see how a person experiencing persecutory delusions could build this reaction into their delusional belief system. It requires urgent action which

is usually the intramuscular or intravenous administration of an antimuscarinic drug such as procyclidine. The dose of procyclidine would usually be 5–10 mg injected intramuscularly, repeated after 20 minutes if recovery does not occur. It can also be given as 5 mg intravenously, in which case recovery would usually be within five minutes. High potency antipsychotics, like haloperidol, are more likely to lead to EPSEs than low potency drugs like thioridazine. Other EPSEs include pseudoparkinsonism which should be treated acutely with an anticholinergic, which can be withdrawn in the longer term in the majority of patients, and akathisia, which may respond to propranolol or cyproheptadine (Weiss et al, 1995). Tardive dyskinesia and neuroleptic malignant syndrome are also likely to be mediated through central dopamine blockade, although relative incidences for individual drugs are difficult to determine.

3. What are the main measures used to assess the side-effects of antipsychotics and what are their strengths and weaknesses?
Table 1 lists the main measures that are available to assess side-effects of antipsychotic medication. The most widely used of these are the Simpson

Table 1
Assessment tools for antipsychotic side effects

Author	Year	Type of side-effect	Number of items
Simpson and Angus	1970	EPSE	10
NIMH AIMS	1980	Dyskinesia	12
Lingjaerde et al UKU	1987	All	48
Barnes	1989	Akathisia	3
Day et al LUNSERS	1995	All	41 + 10 red herrings

EPSE, extrapyramidal side-effects; NIMH, National Institute of Mental Health; AIMS, Abnormal Involuntary Movements Scale; UKU, Scandinavian Society of Psychopharmacology Committee of Clinical Investigations

and Angus scale, which assesses extrapyramidal side-effects, and the Abnormal Involuntary Movement Scale (AIMS), which assesses dyskinesias. These scales have been used in research for many years. They include physical manipulation of the patient and are rather narrow as they focus only on extrapyramidal side-effects. Barnes (1989) developed and validated a scale assessing the severity of akathisia which included subscales of psychological and motor restlessness. The UKU scale has been validated with the use in thousands of patients prescribed antipsychotics and is comprehensive, covering psychic, autonomic, hormonal and allergic side-effects and weight gain, as well as the

extrapyramidal side-effects. The UKU scale includes a rating of the likely causal relationship between the side-effect and the medication. However, this scale is intended to be administered by a trained physician and can take up to an hour to carry out. The Liverpool University Neuroleptic Side Effects Rating Scale (LUNSERS) is based on the UKU, but is self-administered by the patient and therefore can be carried out in approximately 5 to 20 minutes.

4. What syndrome could be responsible for the lack of motivation experienced by MB and how is it best managed?
Neuroleptic-induced deficit syndrome (NIDS) may be responsible. This

syndrome comprises a lack of volition and motivation as well as restricted emotions, inability to think straight and reduced spontaneity (Naber, 1995) and can result in a lowered quality of life, poor compliance and poor outcome in schizophrenia (Lewander, 1994). It is not widely recognised. Also, definitions vary and it is difficult to differentiate between NIDS and the primary negative symptoms of schizophrenia. Management of this side-effect is difficult and there is no good evidence regarding the differential prevalence with different drugs. However, less sedative drugs such as trifluoperazine, haloperidol or sulpiride may be seen as more favourable than the more sedative drugs such as chlorpromazine and thioridazine. It has been suggested that the incidence of NIDS may be lower with the newer atypical antipsychotics, particularly clozapine (although this needs substantiation) (Naber, 1995). With the older drugs, dose reduction may also be helpful, although this should always be slow and the patient carefully monitored for signs of relapse.

Key points

- All antipsychotics have unique side-effect profiles. Non-tolerance of one drug because of a specific side-effect should lead to the choice of another drug with a different side-effect profile.
- Extrapyramidal side-effects are frequently encountered with the older drugs. However, the newer atypical drugs are not without side-effects, some of which (such as weight gain) are distressing, and some (such as agranmocytosis with clozapine) are potentially fatal.
- Several side-effect rating scales are available, although the majority focus on EPSEs. The UKU and LUNSERS include a wider range of items.
- The definition of neuroleptic-induced deficit syndrome includes a lack of volition and motivation, restricted emotions, decreased quality of life, poor compliance and poor outcome. It has been suggested that prevalence of this syndrome may be lower with the new atypical drugs than the older alternatives. However, this needs confirmation.

References

Barnes TRE (1989) A rating scale for drug induced akathisia, *Br J Psychiatry* **154:** 672–6.

Day JC, Wood G, Dewey M et al (1995) A self-rating scale for neuroleptic side effects: validation in a group of schizophrenia patients, *Br J Psychiatry* **166:** 650–3.

Kotin J, Wilber DE, Verburg D (1976) Thioridazine and sexual dysfunction, *Am J Psychiatry* **133:** 82–5.

Lewander T (1994) Neuroleptics and the neuroleptic-induced deficit syndrome, *Acta Psychiatr Scand* **89:** 8–13.

Lingjaerde O, Ahlfors VG, Dech P et al (1987) The UKU side effect rating scale for psychotropic drugs and a cross sectional study of side effects in neuroleptic treated patients, *Acta Psychiatr Scand (Suppl)* **334:** 76.

Munetz MR, Benjamine S (1988) How to examine patients using the Abnormal Involuntary Movements Scale, *Hosp Community Psychiatry* **39:** 1772–7.

Naber D (1995) A self-rating scale to measure subjective effects of neuroleptic drugs, relationships to objective psychopathology, quality of life, compliance and other clinical variables, *Int Clin Psychopharmacol* **10:** (Suppl. 3) 133–8.

Simpson GM, Angus JWS (1970) A rating scale for extra-pyramidal side effects, *Acta Psychiatr Scand* (Suppl) **212:** 11–19.

Sullivan G, Lukoff D (1990) Sexual side effects of antipsychotic medication: evaluation and interventions, *Hosp Community Psychiatry* **41:** 1238–41.

Weiss D, Aizenberg D, Hermesh H (1995) Cyproheptadine treatment in neuroleptic-induced akathisia, *Br J Psychiatry* **167:** 483–6.

Treatment of psychosis in pregnancy and breastfeeding

Robyn McAskill and Ann Hutton

9

AB, a 28-year-old woman, was admitted to hospital because of a deterioration in her mental state. She believed that she was pregnant and was expressing paranoid delusions that her partner was trying to harm her and her baby. On examination, AB had poor eye contact, was extremely suspicious of the ward staff and was seen talking quietly to herself while alone. AB was unkempt, very thin and showed other signs of self-neglect. She did not express any suicidal ideation, nor were there signs of self-harm. AB did not know when she had her last menstrual period (LMP).

Her partner reported that there had been a gradual decline in AB's self-care, that she had not been sleeping well and was very irritable with him. Over the past two to three weeks, AB had accused him of trying to harm her and had often locked him out of their flat. He also reported that six months ago they had decided to have a baby. They discussed it with AB's consultant who agreed to prescribe chlorpromazine instead of her usual depot. AB stopped taking her tablets, probably about four months ago, as they were making her tired and because she feared that the medication would harm her baby.

AB had been diagnosed six years ago as having paranoid schizophrenia. She has had two relapses since then, secondary to non-compliance with oral antipsychotic medication (first haloperidol, then trifluoperazine). During her last admission, three years ago, AB was prescribed Depixol (Flupenthixol decanoate) 40 mg every four weeks and procyclidine 5 mg twice a day. Since then AB has remained well on medication.

AB was willing to stay in hospital but did not want to take any medication as 'it will deform my baby'.

A provisional diagnosis of a relapse of a schizophrenic illness was made. A pregnancy test was positive. An ultrasound scan confirmed that AB was approximately nine weeks pregnant.

Questions

1. How should psychosis in pregnancy be managed?
2. Should antipsychotics be continued through labour and delivery?
3. Should AB breastfeed her baby while taking an antipsychotic?
4. Can antipsychotics cause long-term effects on the infant?

Answers

1. How should psychosis in pregnancy be managed?

When prescribing psychotropics to women of childbearing age it is important to discuss the potential effects of both medication and untreated illness on the unborn child and the mother.

Advice on family planning should be offered.

It is not clear whether psychotic illness is exacerbated or improved during pregnancy. Also, controversy surrounds the question as to whether babies born to women with psychoses are at increased risk of malformations independent of drug exposure (Lee and Donaldson, 1995; Miller 1991).

The pattern of illness experienced by AB is common, with relapses related to non-compliance. AB had discussed her wish to become pregnant with her doctor, but then stopped her oral medication partly because it was making her tired. She and her partner also thought it may harm their baby. Partners may influence a decision regarding medication use in pregnancy, and so it is important that they have a full understanding of the risks of illness and treatment as stated above. Understandably, women may feel a strong sense of determination not to harm their unborn child (Altshuler et al, 1996).

On admission, AB was not sure when her LMP had been. Many antipsychotics cause hyperprolactinaemia which may lead to ammenorrhoea and galactorrhoea in some patients. Ammenorrhoeic women are unlikely to be fertile, although conception is not unknown. It is important to educate women about these adverse effects, as they may lead to unfounded fears of pregnancy. Moreover, without education, some women with major mental illness may be unaware of a pregnancy until it is well advanced. If pregnancy is suspected, it should be confirmed as soon as possible by taking the patient's menstrual history and a urine sample or serum beta-HCG assay for a pregnancy test. Note that some antipsychotics may produce false-positives in some urine pregnancy tests (Miller, 1991). Physical examination and abdominal ultrasound can then be used, if required, to confirm the pregnancy and estimate gestational age.

It was confirmed that AB is pregnant and she has a provisional diagnosis of a relapse of a schizophrenic illness. At this point the clinician and patient are faced with the difficult task of weighing up the risks of medication during pregnancy against the risks of withholding medication. Obviously, psychotropic medication should only be prescribed where the benefits to the mother and child are considered to outweigh the risks.

AB shows signs of self-neglect, paranoid ideation and impulsive behaviour. Untreated symptoms of psychoses can pose a risk to the mother and fetus. Risks include the mother being less able to gain access to prenatal care and make realistic plans for her baby; being more vulnerable to the effects of poor judgement; being less likely to be well nourished; and being more likely to carry out impulsive behaviours including suicide and infanticide (Miller, 1991). The possible impact of untreated symptoms on maternal attachment and child development should also be noted. It is important to consider the patient's previous history together with her insight, social supports and therapeutic alliances. Non-pharmacological treatments such as counselling or psychotherapy should be considered. Organic causes should be excluded.

The main aims of treating AB's relapse include symptom reduction and improving her ability to function so that she is best able to care for herself during pregnancy. Antipsychotics may pose risks during pregnancy as they all cross the placenta freely. Risks include teratogenicity (following first-trimester exposure), neonatal toxicity (if administered close to delivery) and, possibly, more subtle long-term neurobehavioural effects on children and even adults (Trixler and Tenyi, 1997). It should be noted that there are few good quality data on psychotropic agents in pregnancy. Published studies are old, have methodological flaws and give conflicting results. Most larger studies describe outcomes when older antipsychotics in low doses have been used as antiemetics in the first trimester. Although there are a number of case reports of malformation, including multiple anomalies, no clustering has emerged and there may have been confounding factors in these cases (Lee and Donaldson, 1995; Miller, 1991). Most large observational studies have concluded that women who take antipsychotics during pregnancy are at no higher risk of having a deformed child than women who do not.

Of all the antipsychotics, there are most data on the safety of phenothiazines in pregnancy, particularly chlorpromazine and trifluoperazine, and for this reason these antipsychotics are recommended (Lee and Donaldson, 1995). There is relatively little information on the butyrophenones such as haloperidol, despite their widespread use (Lee and Donaldson, 1995; Altshuler et al, 1996). There are very few data on other antipsychotics, particularly the atypicals, and therefore these agents should be avoided. Depots should also be avoided because of their prolonged action (making it difficult to adjust doses) and relatively high incidence of adverse effects (Lee and Donaldson, 1995; Miller, 1991).

Occasionally depots may be required to ensure compliance but other methods should be tried to achieve this.

Some authors advocate the preferential use of high-potency agents because low-potency antipsychotics such as chlorpromazine may cause orthostatic hypotension, sedation, tachycardia, urinary retention and gastrointestinal slowing. These are theoretical considerations only and there is no evidence of improved outcome with high-potency drugs (Lee and Donaldson, 1995).

When evaluating the risks of medication in AB, it can perhaps be concluded that these are smaller than the risks of untreated illness. AB had found chlorpromazine too sedating. She had responded well to trifluoperazine in the past and so trifluoperazine 5 mg bd was prescribed. This was increased to 5 mg tds after a few days and her symptoms began to resolve after two weeks. In general, the minimum effective antipsychotic dose should always be used and the patient's progress monitored with a recognised rating scale such as the Brief Psychiatric Rating Scale (BPRS).

Adverse effects should be regularly assessed. There are few data on the effects of medications used to treat antipsychotic-induced extrapyramidal side-effects (EPSE) in pregnancy. Diphenhydramine (used in the United States) and anticholinergics have been associated with teratogenicity and therefore should be avoided at least in the first trimester. Anticholinergics can also compound the decreased gastrointestinal motility frequently seen in pregnancy. If EPSE do develop, dosage reduction or switching to a low potency agent should be tried first. If a drug is still required to treat EPSE, there is no preferred agent (Miller, 1991; Altshuler et al, 1996).

Maintenance treatment should be considered once AB's symptoms have resolved. Again, the risks and benefits of maintenance therapy should be considered. Obviously drug discontinuation before or during pregnancy may put the patient at risk of relapse. Maintenance antipsychotics before and during pregnancy should be considered in patients with a history of chronic psychoses and in particular those with a history of repeated episodes caused by drug tapering or non-compliance. Maintenance medication may minimise overall fetal exposure by limiting the need for acute treatment with higher doses of medication, should relapse occur.

2. Should antipsychotics be continued through labour and delivery?

The effects of antipsychotic medication on labour and delivery have not been extensively studied. Single doses of antipsychotics have often been given to reduce anxiety during labour (Robinson et al, 1986) but these drugs can cause postural hypotension and cardiac arrhythmias. Because of the effects of labour on the cardiovascular system, these adverse effects are relatively more important. Also, because antipsychotics lower the seizure threshold, there may also be an increased risk of the consequences of eclampsia (Miller, 1991).

The possibility that the mother may have an elective or emergency caesarean section should be considered. In surgery, hypotensive reactions, cardiac arrhythmias and prolonged sedation have been reported when antipsychotics are given before anaesthesia (Stockley, 1996).

Pharmacokinetic interactions between antipsychotics and opiates, muscle relaxants and general anaesthetics, are not well understood. The inhaled general anaesthetics are metabolised in the liver via CYP2E1 (Naguib et al, 1997). Since most of the typical antipsychotics are metabolised via CYP2D6 (Naguib et al, 1997), the risk of significant pharmacokinetic interactions between these drugs is probably small. Reported interactions are most likely to be pharmacodynamic (e.g. sedative, hypotensive and cardiac effects) (Stockley, 1996; Naguib et al, 1997).

When antipsychotics are continued throughout the third trimester, adverse effects in the newborn have been reported. Antipsychotic discontinuation symptoms may occur. These usually present as behavioural effects such as inconsolable crying, agitation and increased sucking (Robinson et al, 1986; Lee and Cohen, 1989; Lee and Donaldson, 1995). Discontinuation symptoms may take three days to appear after birth (Lee and Donaldson, 1995). Other adverse effects reported include: neonatal jaundice, constipation, respiratory depression, melanin deposition in the eyes and extrapyramidal effects (Stowe and Nemeroff, 1995; Miller, 1991; Simpson et al, 1981).

Some authors recommend slowly withdrawing antipsychotic medication two to four weeks before the expected delivery date to prevent the adverse effects mentioned above. However, this may put the mother at risk of recurrence of mental illness. There is also the added risk of puerperal psychosis (Lee and Donaldson, 1995). It is estimated that 50% of women with a previous history of psychosis develop puerperal psychosis.

The effect of puerperal psychosis in the mother on the developing infant is a cause for concern. It is worth noting, should relapse occur, that the mother and baby may be exposed to much higher doses of antipsychotic drugs, since higher doses tend to be used in acute illness.

With respect to AB, it would be prudent to continue her trifluoperazine during labour and delivery, in view of her history of relapse from antipsychotic withdrawal. These issues will need to be discussed with AB and her partner, ideally after her mental state has stabilised. The midwife, obstetrician and anaesthetist (if applicable) should be informed that AB is taking trifluoperazine and the reasons for her continuing it throughout pregnancy. After the birth, AB and her partner need to monitor the baby for adverse effects. AB herself will also need monitoring for signs of recurrence of psychosis (even though she is taking

antipsychotic medication). If available, involvement by a specialist mother and baby Community Psychiatric Nurse (CPN) would be useful. AB's general practitioner and health visitor will also need to be informed that AB is taking trifluoperazine and that adverse effects may develop in the baby.

3. Should AB breastfeed her baby while taking an antipsychotic?

It is widely accepted that, during the first six months of life, breast-milk, compared with infant formulas, provides better nutritional and immunological support for the developing baby. For both the mother and baby there are also psychological benefits to be gained from breastfeeding; it has been shown to assist mother–infant bonding (Buist et al, 1990; Briggs et al, 1994). The general public are very much aware of the advantages of breastfeeding; 42% of mothers continue to breastfeed their babies after the first six weeks of life (Mason, 1998).

All antipsychotics diffuse into breast-milk (Buist et al, 1990). This is probably because of their high lipid solubility but may also be because of protein-binding, although this is less well understood (Briggs et al, 1994). The baby is at risk of experiencing adverse effects from relatively small amounts of antipsychotic taken in during breastfeeding. Antipsychotic drugs bind to albumin and are largely metabolised by the liver. A newborn, full-term baby has an immature liver, reduced blood albumin concentration and an underdeveloped blood–brain barrier (Chisholm and Kuller, 1997). If the baby is premature, adverse effects are thus perhaps even more likely to occur.

Acute and chronic adverse effects in the baby have not been firmly linked to antipsychotic use during breastfeeding. Some information is available as case reports, but this is often conflicting (Maitra and Menkes, 1996). Adverse effects reported in the baby include: drowsiness, lethargy and extrapyramidal effects (Chisholm and Kuller, 1997; Maitra and Menkes, 1996; Robinson et al 1986).

The decision as to whether AB breastfeeds her baby is a difficult one. The benefits of breastfeeding are well established and continuation of antipsychotic medication, in AB's case, is desirable. However, with respect to the baby, the acute and chronic effects of antipsychotic exposure via breast-milk are largely unknown. In this situation,

ideally, the clinician should discuss all risks (known and unknown) with AB and her partner and agree a decision before the start of breastfeeding (ideally before delivery). The overall health of the baby also needs to be considered. If the baby is premature, underweight, has any congenital illness (e.g. cardiovascular malformation), or perinatal complication (e.g. neonatal jaundice), advice from a paediatrician should be sought.

If it is decided that AB will continue her antipsychotic medication and breastfeed her baby, her GP, CPN, midwife and health visitor need to be informed. To minimise the amount of antipsychotic to which the baby is exposed, trifluoperazine should be given as tablets (not sustained-release capsules) as a single dose at night after the last feed. Overnight, AB should be counselled to feed her baby with previously expressed milk or infant formula. This ensures that the baby is not breastfed when the amount of antipsychotic drug in the breast-milk is highest. AB and her partner also need to be given some guidance on what adverse effects are possible in the baby and how to manage them (the CPN and health visitor could assist them with this). They also need to understand the importance of child health clinic visits to monitor the overall health and development of the child.

4. Can antipsychotics cause long-term effects on the infant?

In animal studies, fetal exposure to antipsychotics can affect vasculogenesis, neurogenesis, central catecholamine levels and dopamine receptor function. There are conflicting reports of persistent abnormalities in learning behaviour (Kerns, 1986). The extent to which these data can be extrapolated to humans is unclear.

Surprisingly, there is little research regarding neurobehavioural effects from fetal exposure to antipsychotics. Without continuous follow-up, it is impossible to estimate emotional, cognitive and behavioural effects in children who were exposed to antipsychotics in the womb.

Following several case reports of persistent neurobehavioural abnormalities in children, a few larger studies have been published. Two studies (cited in Trixler and Tenyi, 1997) followed children up to the age of five years and found no difference in behavioural and intellectual functioning in those exposed in utero to low-dose pheno-

thiazines compared with controls. In another controlled study, 68 children exposed to antipsychotics in the second half of pregnancy had their behaviour at school examined. No statistical differences from controls were found (cited in Trixler and Tenyi, 1997). A further study of 151 children exposed to phenothiazines during pregnancy found no difference in IQ scores at four years compared with controls (cited in Kerns, 1986).

These studies represent small samples, generally exposed to low doses of phenothiazines at variable times of pregnancy. Better controlled, more rigorous follow-up studies are needed to draw firm conclusions. Caution is advised.

Key points

- The potential effects of both medication and untreated illness on the unborn child and the mother should be considered.
- Risks include teratogenicity (when taken in the first trimester), neonatal toxicity (if taken up to delivery) and possibly long-term neurobehavioural effects.
- Most large observational studies have concluded that women who

take antipsychotics during pregnancy are at no higher risk of having a malformed child than women who do not.

- There is more clinical experience with chlorpromazine and trifluoperazine and these drugs are generally considered to be safe.
- There are few data available on the atypical drugs.
- Preterm infants (with very immature hepatic metabolising capacity) should probably not be breastfed while the mother is taking antipsychotic drugs.
- Exposure of the breastfed infant to antipsychotics can be minimised by administering the drug to the mother as a single daily dose at night after the last feed.

References

Altshuler LL, Cohen L, Szuba MP et al (1996) Pharmacologic management of psychiatric illness during pregnancy: dilemmas and guidelines, *Am J Psychiatry* **153:** 592–606.

Briggs GG, Freeman RK, Yaffe SJ (1994) *Drugs in Pregnancy and Lactation*, 4th edn. (Baltimore: Maryland: Williams and Wilkins).

Buist A, Norman TR, Dennerstein L (1990) Breastfeeding and the use of psychotropic medication: a review, *J Affect Disord* **19:** 197–206.

Chisholm CA, Kuller JA (1997) A guide to the safety of CNS-active agents during breastfeeding, *Drug Safety* **17:** 127–42.

Kerns LL (1986) Treatment of mental disorders in pregnancy: a review of psychotropic drug risks and benefits, *J Nerv Ment Dis* **174:** 652–9.

Lee A, Donaldson S (1995) Drug use in pregnancy: psychiatric and neurological disorders: part 1, *Pharm J* **254:** 87–90.

Cohen LS (1989) Psychotropic drug use in pregnancy, *Hosp Community Psychiatry* **40:** 566–7.

Maitra R, Menkes DB (1996) Psychotropic drugs and lactation, *NZ Med J* **109:** 217–19.

Mason P (1998) Infant feeding – an update, *Pharm J* **260:** 51–4.

Miller LJ (1991) Clinical strategies for the use of psychotropic drugs during pregnancy, *Psychiatr Med* **9:** 275–97.

Naguib M, Magboul MA, Jaroudi R (1997) Clinically significant drug interactions with general anaesthetics, *CNS Drugs* **8:** 51–78.

Robinson GE, Stewart DE, Flak E (1986) The rational use of psychotropic drugs in pregnancy and postpartum, *Can J Psychiatry* **31:** 183–90.

Simpson GM, Pi EH, Sramek Jr JJ (1981) Adverse effects of antipsychotic agents, *Drugs* **21:** 138–51.

Stockley IH (1996) *Drug Interactions* (Oxford: Blackwell Scientific Publications).

Stowe ZN, Nemeroff CB (1995) Psychopharmacology during pregnancy and lactation. In: Schatzberg AF, Nemeroff CB, eds. *Textbook of Psychopharmacology.* (Washington DC: American Psychiatric Press) 823–37.

Trixler M, Tenyi T (1997) Antipsychotic use in pregnancy: what are the best treatment options? *Drug Safety* **16:** 403–10.

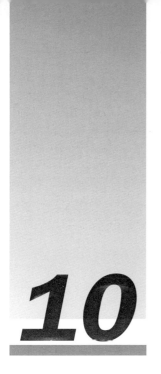

Treatment of psychosis in people with epilepsy

Denise Duncan

10

RT, a 28-year-old Caucasian man with a 14-year history of refractory complex–partial seizures was brought to hospital by the police. He had threatened his mother with a knife because he believed she was collaborating with aliens to poison him. Mental state examination revealed auditory hallucinations, thought insertion and thought blocking, delusions of persecution and loosening of associations. He was admitted to hospital and prescribed chlorpromazine 250 mg four times a day. He was later diagnosed as having a schizophrenia-like psychosis of epilepsy.

Medications on admission:

Vigabatrin	2000 mg bd (for last six months)
Valproate	500 mg bd (10 years)
Carbamazepine	200 mg bd (1 year)

Over the following month it was noted that RT was having up to five seizures a week.

Lamotrigine was started at 25 mg/day and increased to 50 mg after two weeks and then 100 mg two weeks later. RT's seizures improved, his psychosis resolved and he was discharged. Two weeks later the patient presented to the clinic with a maculopapular rash.

Questions

1. What factors contribute to psychosis in people with epilepsy?
2. Which drug is likely to have caused the rash and why?
3. What important factors need to be considered in the treatment of psychosis in people with epilepsy?
4. How could this patient's antiepileptic drug therapy be simplified?

Answers

1. What factors contribute to psychosis in people with epilepsy?

Factors that have been shown to contribute to psychosis, include:

- Polypharmacy
- Complex-partial seizure type
- Male sex
- A long history of seizures (14 years in this patient). (The average onset of psychosis occurring with epilepsy is 12 to 15 years after seizure onset.)
- Vigabatrin and possibly other antiepileptic drugs (AEDS) (McConnell & Duncan, 1998a).

2. Which drug is likely to have caused the rash and why?

The rash is most likely to have been caused by lamotrigine. The temporal association is striking and lamotrigine is well known to cause rash. Rashes associated with lamotrigine are usually described as maculopapular or morbilliform and occur most commonly in the first eight weeks of therapy. Rash has been reported to occur in up to 11.2% of subjects receiving lamotrigine, although the incidence has been as high as 18.7% in patients who were taking both lamotrigine and valproate (Gilman, 1995). More serious skin reactions such as Stevens–Johnson syndrome and toxic epidermal necrolysis occur in only approximately one in every 1000 adults and between one in 300 and one in 100 children (data on file, Glaxo Wellcome). Extreme caution should therefore be exercised.

The development of skin reactions is thought to be related to high initial lamotrigine serum levels. High serum levels are most likely to occur in children or when there are high initial doses. Rapid dose titration or concomitant valproate therapy and possibly a history of drug allergies or an allergy to another AED also make rash more likely. Valproate, a known enzyme inhibitor, inhibits lamotrigine's metabolism and prolongs its half-life from a mean of 29 hours to 60 hours. Conversely, enzyme inducers (e.g. phenytoin, carbamazepine, phenobarbitone), when prescribed with lamotrigine, may reduce its half-life to approximately 15 hours. For these reasons there are three different dosing regimes with lamotrigine therapy. These are monotherapy, prescription with valproate therapy or prescription with enzyme-inducing drugs without valproate. As RT was receiving valproate, his lamotrigine should have been prescribed at a dose of 25 mg every second day for two weeks, then increased to 25 mg every day for two

weeks and then increased by 25–50 mg every one to two weeks, with the usual maintenance dose being 100–200 mg/day. If rapid dosage titration is thought to be responsible for the rash, it is possible to rechallenge the patient successfully if slow dosage titration is subsequently employed.

3. What important factors need to be considered in the treatment of psychosis in people with epilepsy?

Before an antipsychotic is prescribed to someone with epilepsy it must be decided whether or not the psychosis and seizures are related. If there is a temporal relationship between the seizure and psychosis (peri-ictal psychosis, where the psychosis is apparent either during or immediately after the seizure), the patient is best treated by optimising their AED therapy (McConnell & Duncan, 1998b). Such patients should not generally be given antipsychotics (which could potentially further lower their seizure threshold, causing more seizures and consequently more psychosis), although occasionally in post-ictal psychosis (psychosis occurring immediately after a seizure) short-term use of antipsychotics may be necessary.

If the psychosis occurs independently of seizures (inter-ictal psychosis), long-term antipsychotic treatment will probably be necessary. Obviously, when choosing an antipsychotic in people with epilepsy, it is important to take into account what effects the drug has on seizure threshold and whether it is likely to interact with any drugs the patient is taking. Once the drug is chosen, it is then important to start at a low dose and increase slowly. This is because changes in doses during initiation, titration and withdrawal of medication (as well as total dose) may all effect seizure threshold (Itil & Soldatos, 1980).

It appears that chlorpromazine is the phenothiazine antipsychotic most likely to lower seizure threshold. Logothetis (1967), after following 1,528 patients (with no previous history of epilepsy) who were taking phenothiazines for four and half years, found that chlorpromazine had the highest seizure risk, with 9% of those who received more than 1000 mg of chlorpromazine a day developing seizures. Toone & Fenton (1977) also found that seizures were more likely to occur with chlorpromazine (mean dose 266 mg) than with other antipsychotics.

Thioridazine has been suggested as a better choice, as it is said to be less likely to lower the seizure threshold (Remick & Fine, 1987). However, this may be because the maximum dose is 800 mg/day and so relatively smaller doses of the drug tend to be used compared with chlorpromazine. Sudden death occurs not infrequently in epilepsy and because thioridazine has been the antipsychotic most associated with sudden death (Mehtonen et al, 1991), this drug should perhaps be avoided in treating people with epilepsy.

Of the typical antipsychotics, trifluoperazine, fluphenazine, perphenazine and haloperidol are thought to be relatively less likely to lower the seizure threshold (Trimble, 1985; Markowitz & Brown, 1987) and haloperidol has been suggested to be one of the antipsychotics of choice in epilepsy (Fenwick, 1995).

Of the atypical drugs, risperidone and sulpiride may be the drugs of choice. Risperidone was associated with only a 0.3% seizure incidence in clinical trials, while sulpiride appears to have minimal effects on EEG; there have been only two case reports of seizures to the manufacturer, Lorex (McConnell et al, 1997). Conversely, clozapine is the most epileptogenic antipsychotic and its effect on seizure threshold is related to both dose and titration rate. Doses below 300 mg/day are associated with a 1% seizure risk, while doses above 600 mg/day have a seizure risk of 4.4% (Toth & Frakenburg, 1994). There are still too few data available on sertindole, olanzapine and quetiapine to recommend their use in people with epilepsy.

Carbamazepine may lower antipsychotic plasma levels and has been associated with an exacerbation of psychotic symptoms when added to haloperidol (Arana et al, 1986). Conversely, the withdrawal of carbamazepine may increase serum levels, causing extrapyramidal side-effects (Fast et al, 1986). Carbamazepine can also lower serum levels of clozapine, sertindole and olanzapine (Tiihonen et al, 1995; Lundbeck SPC; Lilly SPC), probably through its ability to induce the hepatic metabolising enzyme CYP1A2. Phenytoin, another enzyme inducer, may have similar effects (Miller, 1991).

In conclusion, it appears that clozapine, chlorpromazine and loxapine are more epileptogenic than other antipsychotics and so should be avoided in people with epilepsy. Risperidone, sulpiride and haloperidol appear to be less likely to lower the seizure threshold. Trifluoperazine, fluphenazine and zuclopenthixol are other alternatives. It is important that only one antipsychotic is given at any one time and that treatment should be initiated with a low dose and increased slowly. AED serum levels should be monitored when an antipsychotic is co-prescribed.

4. How could this patient's antiepileptic drug therapy be simplified?

With respect to AED therapy, more drugs rarely equate to better seizure control. As lamotrigine has most probably caused a rash in RT, it should be discontinued. Vigabatrin should also be slowly withdrawn, because of the risk that it may be contributing to RT's psychosis. Because carbamazepine and valproate are likely to be at sub-therapeutic doses, plasma levels should be taken and their doses optimised. If seizures are controlled, consideration should be given to weaning the least effective of these two drugs (ask the patient) over several months. The vast majority of patients are better controlled on mono- or duo-therapy.

Key points

- Factors that contribute to the development of psychosis in people with epilepsy include polypharmacy, having complex-partial seizures, being male, having a long history of seizures and some anticonvulsant drugs such as vigabatrin.

- It is important to determine whether the psychosis is peri-ictal or inter-ictal before embarking on a treatment regimen.
- Peri-ictal psychosis is best treated by optimising anticonvulsant cover.
- Inter-ictal psychosis requires treatment with antipsychotics.
- Haloperidol, sulpiride and risperidone are three of the safest drugs to use in epilepsy.
- Clozapine, chlorpromazine and loxapine are most likely to reduce the seizure threshold.

References

Arana GW, Goff DC, Friedman H et al (1986) Does carbamazepine-induced reduction of plasma haloperidol levels worsen psychotic symptoms? *Am J Psychiatry* **143:** 650–1.

Fast DK, Jones BD, Kusalic M et al (1986) Effect of carbamazepine on neuroleptic plasma levels and efficacy, *Am J Psychiatry* **143:** 117–8.

Fenwick P (1995) Psychiatric disorder and epilepsy. In: Hopkins A, Shorvon S, Cascino G, eds. *Epilepsy*. (London: Chapman & Hall Medical) 453–502.

Gilman JT (1995) Lamotrigine: an anti-epileptic agent for the treatment of partial seizures, *Ann Pharmacother* **29:** 144–51.

Itil TM, Soldatos C (1980) Epileptogenic side effects of psychotropic drugs, *J Am Med Assoc* **244:** 1460–3.

Logothetis J (1967) Spontaneous epileptic seizures and EEG changes in the course of phenothiazine therapy, *Neurology* **17:** 869–77.

Markowitz JC, Brown RP (1987) Seizures with neuroleptics and antidepressants, *Gen Hosp Psychiatry* **9:** 135–41.

McConnell H, Duncan D, Taylor D (1997) Choice of neuroleptics in epilepsy. *Psychiatr Bull* **21:** 642–5.

McConnell HW, Duncan D (1998a) Behavioral effects of antiepileptic drugs. In: McConnell HW, Snyder PJ, eds. *Epilepsy and Psychiatric Comorbidity: Basic Mechanisms, Diagnosis and Treatment.* (Washington DC: American Psychiatric Press) 205–44.

McConnell HW, Duncan D (1998b) Treatment of psychiatric comorbidity in epilepsy. In: McConnell HW, Snyder PJ, eds. *Epilepsy and Psychiatric Comorbidity: Basic Mechanisms, Diagnosis and Treatment.* (Washington DC: American Psychiatric Press) 245–361.

Mehtonen OP, Aranko K, Mälkonen L (1991) A survey of sudden death associated with the use of antipsychotic or antidepressant drugs: 49 cases in Finland, *Acta Psychiatr Scand* **84:** 58–64.

Miller DD (1991) Effect of phenytoin on plasma clozapine concentrations in two patients, *J Clin Psychiatry* **52:** 23–5.

Remick R, Fine S (1979) Antipsychotic drugs and seizures, *J Clin Psychiatry* **40:** 78–80.

Tiihonen J, Vartiainen H, Hakola P (1995) Carbamazepine induced changes in plasma levels of neuroleptics, *Pharmacopsychiatry* **28:** 26–8.

Toone BK, Fenton GW (1977) Epileptic seizures induced by psychotropic drugs, *Psychol Med* **7:** 265–70.

Toth P, Frankenburg FR (1994) Clozapine and seizures – a review, *Can J Psychiatry* **39:** 236–8.

Trimble MR (1985) The psychoses of epilepsy and their treatment. In: Trimble MR, ed. *The Psychopharmacology of Epilepsy.* (Chichester: John Wiley and Sons) 83–94.

Depression with anxiety symptoms

Celia Feetam

FM, a 46-year-old man, was admitted to the psychiatric unit of his local district general hospital. FM had experienced breathlessness and severe palpitations, he had felt hot and sweaty and had almost fainted, and although these feelings had passed quickly, both FM and his wife had been very frightened by the episode and were concerned that he may have had a heart attack.

On admission FM confessed to having felt under considerable pressure for some time. He had not slept properly for weeks, waking early most mornings, and he no longer had a good appetite. He admitted to feeling low, lethargic and lacking in energy and, although once a keen cyclist, FM had not been out on his bike for months, preferring instead to spend his spare time just sitting at home. On further questioning FM said he felt unable to carry on, that 'life was not worth living' and that 'his family would be better off without him'.

When FM left school he had joined the armed forces and seen active service. On discharge he had become a policeman but, although he was very successful and gained rapid promotion, he never liked the work and eventually resigned. He was now in a poorly paid, routine job and had severe financial problems. FM's company had recently relocated to the south of England where he now lived in rented accommodation with his wife and two sons. They had all been reluctant to move and were finding it difficult to settle. His previous medical history was unremarkable. He was taking no regular prescribed medication.

There was no family psychiatric history. FM's parents, although elderly, were alive and well, both physically and mentally. On examination FM appeared thin, tired-looking and somewhat agitated. He did not smoke and drank only very occasionally. Despite his fears that he may have had a heart attack, his ECG was entirely normal, as were his biochemical and haematological results.

Questions

1. What treatment options are available for FM?
2. What factors govern the choice of treatment?
3. What considerations should be given to the way treatment is initiated, continued and, when necessary, eventually discontinued?

Answers

1. What treatment options are available for FM?

This patient is clearly depressed but he is also suffering from anxiety, which in his case is characterised by panic attacks. Up to two-thirds of patients suffering from depression may have associated anxiety symptoms (Clayton et al, 1991). Such anxiety can take the form of psychological or somatic anxiety symptoms, phobias or panic attacks. If depression is the primary condition then its effective treatment should be sufficient in most cases to relieve concomitant anxiety (Coplan and Gorman, 1990).

An antidepressant is clearly indicated for FM. Either a tricyclic or a selective serotonin re-uptake inhibitor may be an appropriate choice at this stage, since certain members of both of these groups of drugs have significant anxiolytic properties in addition to their antidepressant effect (Tyrer and Hallstrom, 1993).

Central serotonin (5HT) system have been implicated in the aetiology of anxiety and panic disorder (Yocca, 1990). Many antidepressants with marked anxiolytic properties inhibit the re-uptake of serotonin in the synaptic cleft. This occurs early in treatment, but like the antidepressant effect of these drugs, anxiolytic effects take some weeks to develop. For the full anxiolytic effect to become apparent, it may be necessary for the $5HT_{1A}$ inhibitory receptors to be desensitised. This occurs only after continued treatment and it is thought to lead to an overall increase in 5HT neurotransmission (Cowen, 1997).

The selective serotonin re-uptake inhibitor paroxetine has been shown to be significantly more effective than placebo in the treatment of panic disorder (Oehrberg et al, 1995) as has citalopram (Wade et al, 1997). Both of these antidepressants are thus licensed for the treatment of panic disorder as well as depression. Fluoxetine, sertraline and nefazodone are all addtionally licensed for the treatment of depression accompanied by anxiety but not for panic disorder.

Of the tricyclics, clomipramine, imipramine or perhaps amitriptyline may be possible options at this stage (Lydiard and Ballenger, 1987). Their anxiolytic effect may be a result of serotonin re-uptake inhibition, or via adrenergic alpha$_2$-autoreceptors.

Since most antidepressants take between four and six weeks to show their full clinical efficacy as either antidepressants or anxiolytics it may also be necessary, in the interim, to prescribe a short course of an additional, faster acting anxiolytic such as a benzodiazepine. This would immediately address the anxiety symptoms, which are likely to be the most troublesome and disabling aspect of the illness for the patient at this time (Cowen, 1997).

2. What factors govern the choice of treatment?
One of the tricyclic group of antidepressants may be the first choice of

treatment for FM, largely because of low cost and proven efficacy. FM does not have cardiac problems. His concerns on this matter were very probably part of the anxiety syndrome and the characteristic somatic symptoms of a panic attack. The tricyclics would be contraindicated if this were not the case because of their cardiotoxicity (Jefferson, 1975). FM is not obese or elderly and therefore less likely to be intolerant of any of the anticholinergic side-effects of a tricyclic compound. However, he has exhibited some suicidal ideation, in which case an older tricyclic agent may be hazardous in view of their toxicity in overdosage (Beaumont, 1989). The Fatal Toxicity Index (FTI) is a means of comparing the potential toxicity in overdosage of antidepressants. It is a measure of the volume of prescribing of a drug in the community together with an estimate of the number of deaths attributed to overdose involving that drug. It is defined as the number of associated deaths per million prescriptions. Amitriptyline, for example, has an FTI of 38.94 (Henry, 1997). Of the new generation, atypical antidepressants, either lofepramine or trazodone, may be safer, as they have FTIs of 2.42 and 7.83, respectively, with trazodone having a slight advan-

tage in FM's case as it is more sedating than lofepramine and may therefore be more suitable for FM, who is agitated and complaining of sleep problems. (Note that FTIs are only rough estimates of toxicity: treatments are not randomly assigned.)

While the relative toxicity in overdose of antidepressants should always be considered when prescribing for an individual patient, it should be noted that, from an epidemiological perspective, there is no evidence that prescribing only the newer drugs will reduce the suicidal rate. Jick et al (1995) followed a cohort of over 170,000 people who had been prescribed antidepressants at least once by their GP, over a five-year period. Although some variables, such as male sex and having received a prescription for an antidepressant in the last 30 days, were found to be associated with completed suicide, the choice of antidepressant was not. Those patients prescribed lofepramine, fluoxetine and trazodone died by violent means or carbon monoxide poisoning rather than overdose.

A selective serotonin re-uptake anti-depressant with anxiolytic properties, such as paroxetine, may, however, be the best choice for FM. Paroxetine, with an FTI of 2.6, would be safe in overdosage, is only mildly sedating and is at least as effective an antidepressant as imipramine (Dunbar et al, 1991). As an interim measure, a long-acting benzodiazepine with active metabolites such as diazepam, could be used on an 'as required' basis for its speed of action and general efficacy in treating the symptoms of panic disorder and anxiety (Nutt, 1996).

If benzodiazepine dependence and withdrawal were a potential cause for concern in FM, a beta-adrenergic blocking agent such as propranolol could be used. These drugs sometimes alleviate the sympathetic symptoms of anxiety such as sweating, tremor, shortness of breath and palpitations, although they are generally considered to be ineffective in reducing most of the psychological manifestations of anxiety (Bailly, 1996).

3. What considerations should be given to the way treatment is initiated, continued and, when necessary, eventually discontinued?

In view of the associated anxiety symptoms, treatment with a selective serotonin re-uptake inhibitor should be initiated cautiously with a low dose, such as 10–20 mg daily of paroxetine, for the first week, together with the chosen short-term anxiolytic agent such as diazepam on an 'as required' basis. This is because an exacerbation of anxiety symptoms and panic frequency is commonly seen during the early stages of treatment with an antidepressant such as paroxetine (Nutt, 1996) and, like the tricyclics, onset of both anxiolytic and antidepressant effect may be delayed for several weeks. Gradual dose titration upwards may be needed to avoid this situation together with careful reassurance of the patient to ensure compliance. Care must be taken to use a therapeutic dose, whichever antidepressant is prescribed.

Treatment at the full, optimum, effective dose, which in view of the associated anxiety syndrome is likely to be at the higher end of the scale for the treatment of a major depression, should continue for at least six months from when a remission of symptoms first occurs (British Association of Psychopharmacology, 1993).

When the decision to discontinue treatment is made it should be done cautiously with a gradual reduction of dosage over a period of two to four weeks (or longer if necessary) to avoid discontinuation symptoms such as dizziness, sensory disturbances, sleep disturbances, agitation or anxiety, nausea, sweating and confusion (Coupland et al, 1996). In respect of the SSRIs, such symptoms are thought to arise as a result of the prolonged desensitisation of the $5HT_{1A}$ inhibitory receptors. When the antidepressant is discontinued, the concentration of serotonin may be insufficient to produce an adequate stimulus for these subsensitive receptors. Discontinuation symptoms have also been reported to occur when tricyclic antidepressants, or indeed antidepressants from any class, are discontinued abruptly. The symptom profile and receptor mechanism differs between individual drugs. Withdrawal from paroxetine can be particularly troublesome. The dose should be slowly reduced, usually over a month or more.

Key points

- Up to two-thirds of depressed patients have co-morbid anxiety symptoms.
- If depression is the primary diagnosis, antidepressants should treat the associated anxiety symptoms.
- SSRIs and tricyclic antidepressants are effective treatments, taking four to six weeks to reach their optimal effect.

- Slow dosage titration may be required to prevent a temporary increase in anxiety symptoms.
- Immediate relief may be obtained by the short-term use of benzodiazepines.
- Treatment should continue for at least six months after recovery, to prevent early relapse.
- Antidepressant doses should be titrated downwards at the end of the treatment period to avoid discontinuation symptoms.

References

Bailly D (1996) The role of beta-adrenoreceptor blockers in the treatment of psychiatric disorders, *CNS Drugs* **5:** 110–23.

Beaumont G (1989) The toxicity of antidepressants, *Br J Psychiatry* **154:** 454–58.

British Association of Psychopharmacology (1993) Guidelines for treating depressive illness with antidepressants, *J Psychopharmacol* **7:** 19–23.

Clayton PJ, Grove WM, Coryell W et al (1991) Follow-up and family study of anxious depression, *Am J Psychiatry* **148:** 1512–17.

Coplan JD, Gorman MJ (1990) Treatment of anxiety disorder in patients with affective disorders, *J Clin Psychiatry* **51:** (Suppl.), 10.

Coupland NJ, Bell C, Potokar J (1996) Serotonin re-uptake inhibitor withdrawal, *J Psychopharmacol* **16:** 356–62.

Cowen PJ (1997) Pharmacotherapy for anxiety disorders: drugs available, *Adv Psychiatr Treat* **3:** 66–7.

Dunbar GC, Cohn JB, Fabre LF et al (1991) A comparison of paroxetine, imipramine and placebo in depressed outpatients, *Br J Psychiatry* **159:** 394–8.

Henry JA (1997) Epidemiology and relative toxicity of antidepressant drugs in overdosage, *Drug Soc* **16:** 375–89.

Jefferson JW (1975) A review of the cardio-vascular effects and toxicity of tricyclic antidepressants, *Pyschosom Med* **37:** 160–78.

Jick SS, Dean AD, Jick H (1995) Antidepressants and suicide, *Br Med J* **310:** 215–18.

Lydiard RB, Ballenger JC (1987) Anti-depressants in panic disorder and agora-phobia, *J Affect Disord* **13:** 153–68.

Nutt DJ (1996) The psychopharmacology of anxiety, *J Hosp Med* **55:** 187–90.

Oehrberg S, Christiansen PE, Behnke K et al (1995) Paroxetine in the treatment of panic disorder. A randomised, double-blind, placebo controlled study, *Br J Psychiatry* **167:** 374–9.

Tyrer P, Hallstrom C (1993) Antidepressants in the treatment of anxiety disorder, *Psychiatr Bull* **16:** 75–6.

Wade AG, Lepola U, Koponen HJ et al (1997) The effect of citalopram in panic disorder, *Br J Psychiatry* **170:** 549–53.

Yocca FD (1990) Neurochemistry and neuro-physiology of buspirone and gepirone: inter-actions of pre-synaptic and post-synaptic $5HT_{1A}$ receptors, *J Clin Psychopharmacol* (Suppl. 3), 6S-12S.

Panic disorder

Celia Feetam

12

TF, a 30-year-old male architect, was admitted to a psychiatric unit following an outpatient consultation with his psychiatrist.

TF had a long history of generalised anxiety disorder (GAD) with panic attacks, and had had several previous admissions. His last admission was some four years earlier when he responded well to imipramine, group therapy and anxiety management.

On admission, TF was clearly extremely anxious. There were no psychotic symptoms and his memory and intellect were both intact. All aspects of a physical examination were entirely normal except for a raised but regular pulse. All biochemistry and haematology tests were also normal. There was no history of any relevant past physical illness. Both his ECG and EEG were normal. He neither smoked nor drank significantly.

For several months before this admission TF had been reasonably well maintained on:

S.R.Propranolol	80 mg daily
Sertraline	50 mg daily
Diazepam	10 mg three times a day.

This regimen had reduced the frequency of his panic attacks but there had always been a background anxiety which had increased significantly over the past three to four weeks to the extent that he now found it difficult to concentrate or to function normally.

TF complained of always feeling low and agitated. He had been hyperventilating and suffered severe palpitations with the result that he was no longer able to work and rarely left his home. His speech was rapid and garbled. He was breathless at rest and at exercise and demonstrated vasomotor lability.

On admission the propranolol and sertraline were stopped abruptly but the diazepam was continued at the same dosage.

In view of the duration and severity of his symptoms and his previous drug history it was decided to try a mono-amine oxidase inhibitor

(MAOI). Phenelzine 15 mg twice a day was prescribed. After three days there was a small but encouraging early improvement and so the dose of phenelzine was increased to 15 mg three times a day.

After two further weeks there was no further improvement. TF continued to experience occasional severe panic attacks every three to four days with attacks of lesser severity intervening. His speech remained rapid and garbled and he continued to look tense. He still tended to avoid stressful situations.

The decision was made to reduce the diazepam and to introduce sodium valproate at a dose of 200 mg three times a day. After a week TF was subjectively improved. His panic attacks reduced in both severity and frequency. During the following week he continued to make good progress and was discharged.

It was decided that he should continue to attend the hospital three times a week as a day patient and undergo cognitive behavioural therapy. He would take the medication as prescribed with a continued gradual reduction of the diazepam.

Questions

1. What pharmacological treatment options are available for the treatment of panic disorder? Briefly outline the differences between them.
2. What is the likely mechanism of action of these drugs?
3. Comment on the drug therapy used in this case.
4. Comment on the abrupt discontinuation of sertraline in this case.

Answers

1. What pharmacological treatment options are available for the treatment of panic disorder? Briefly outline the differences between them.

In general only short-term benefit is to be gained from drug treatment alone. Relapse rates are high within months of stopping medication, so long-term treatment or combination therapy may be necessary.

Panic attacks are usually followed by avoidance behaviour. The optimum strategy would be to suppress the symptoms of panic pharmacologically and then to modify behaviour and cognition with cognitive behavioural therapy. There is increasing evidence for the efficacy of cognitive behavioural therapy in panic disorder (Sharp et al, 1996).

Tricyclic antidepressants, mono-amine oxidase inhibitors and selective serotonin re-uptake inhibitors as well as benzodiazepines have all been shown to be effective pharmacological treatments for panic disorders although their spectrum of activity is different (Liebowitz, 1989). It has long been known that benzodiazepines block anticipatory anxiety, whereas antidepressants prevent panic attacks but, at least initially, not anticipatory anxiety (Klein, 1964). Diazepam, chlordiazepoxide, alprazolam and clonazepam have all been used to provide short-term relief from symptoms until antidepressants have time to exert their effects (Liebowitz, 1989).

Benzodiazepines are usually effective for the first week or more, but tolerance invariably develops. A worsening of symptoms can occur on withdrawal of treatment and this can lead to continuation of therapy with ensuing longer-term problems. (The short-acting benzodiazepine alprazolam has been tentatively shown to be the quickest, most effective treatment, with clonazepam also showing some efficacy (Cross National Collaborative Panic Study, 1992)).

Antidepressants can take from four to six weeks to show maximum efficacy and some have also been shown to produce an increase in anxiety symptoms during the first weeks of treatment which may lead to poor compliance. It is important to start treatment with low doses (e.g. imipramine 10–25 mg/day) and increase slowly to minimise side-effects (Aronson, 1987)). Tolerance does not develop to their beneficial effects and they do not produce dependence. The tricyclics and monoamine oxidase inhibitors do, of course, have some troublesome side-effects, adverse reactions and potential drug interactions. In particular the mono-amine oxidase inhibitors can give rise to serious reactions with tyramine-containing foods. In contrast, moclobemide, a reversible and selective inhibitor of mono-amine oxidase type A only, lacks any significant interaction with food, at least at low doses, and is said to have a quicker onset of action (Priest,

1990), although this claim is not widely accepted.

Of the tricyclics, imipramine and clomipramine seem to be the most effective with clomipramine being superior (Modigh et al, 1992). Controlled studies of the selective serotonin re-uptake inhibitors show that paroxetine (Oehrberg et al, 1995; Ballenger et al, 1998), citalopram (Wade et al, 1997) and fluvoxamine (Hoehn-Saric et al, 1993) are all effective although to date only paroxetine and citalopram have been licensed for use in panic disorder. Benefit has also been demonstrated with the mono-amine oxidase inhibitor phenelzine although this is an unlicensed use for this drug.

Despite initial claims to the contary, (Gastfriend and Rosenbaum, 1989) buspirone, a partial agonist at $5HT_{1A}$ receptors and chemically unrelated to any other anxiolytic, would seem to be ineffective in panic disorder even with higher doses of the order of 60 mg/day (Sheehan et al, 1993).

The evidence for the efficacy of beta-adrenergic blocking agents in panic disorder is equivocal. Some workers have shown a combination of propranolol and a benzodiazepine to be beneficial while others have suggested that it is no better then placebo in this condition (Bailly, 1996). Nevertheless, there seems to be little doubt that this group of drugs has a significant effect on the somatic symptoms of anxiety. In particular it has been shown that propranolol is of value in the treatment of hyperventilation (Suzman, 1971). They are not, however, without side-effects – fatigue and sexual dysfunction being commonly reported (Kostis, 1990).

Although unlicensed for this indication, there is some evidence of the efficacy of sodium valproate in the treatment of panic disorder (Woodmen and Noyes, 1994). Double-blind studies are still required for further verification of these findings.

One interesting double-blind, placebo-controlled, cross-over trial found inositol (an isomer of glucose) to be effective in the treatment of panic disorder. Efficacy was particularly high in the subset of patients who experienced ten or more panic attacks per week at baseline (Benjamin et al, 1995).

2. What is the likely mechanism of action of these drugs?
Central noradrenergic, serotonin, dopaminergic and GABA transmission systems have all been implicated in the aetiology of anxiety states. The benzodiazepines are thought to exert their action on the GABA receptor, mimicking the action of the inhibitory transmitter gamma-aminobutyric acid (Nutt, 1992). Similarly, sodium valproate appears to mimic the action of the benzodiazepines in this respect (Roy-Burne et al, 1989).

It has been postulated that the SSRIs and clomipramine exert their anxiolytic effects via the serotonin system by increasing the overall level of central serotonergic transmission by inhibiting serotonin re-uptake and by a direct desensitising effect on pre- and post-synaptic inhibitory $5HT_{1A}$ receptors (Cowen, 1997).

Noradrenergic antidepressants such as imipramine may exert their antipanic effect via presynaptic adrenergic $alpha_2$-autoreceptors (interfering with the negative feedback mechanism) (Heninger and Charney, 1988). Adrenergic $alpha_2$-receptors are also found on presynaptic serotonin neurones.

Whilst the beta-blockers predominantly affect the peripheral somatic symptoms of anxiety it is thought possible that another important mechanism of action of the more lipophylic compounds is an interaction with central 5HT receptors along with beta-adrenergic blockade in the brain stem (Bailly, 1996).

Inositol is required for the functioning of the phosphatidyl-inositol cycle, a second messenger system used by some serotonergic and adrenergic pathways (Benjamin et al, 1995).

3. Comment on the drug therapy used in this case.

The selective serotonin re-uptake inhibitor sertraline is perhaps not the most effective of this group of antidepressants in reducing the symptoms of panic disorder although it is licensed for the treatment of depression accompanied by anxiety. A higher dose of sertraline, to a maximum of 200 mg a day, could have been tried before the drug was discontinued. Similarly, the dose of phenelzine could have been titrated upwards, side-effects permitting, to a maximum of 105 mg per day. In addition to this, up to 1000 mg per day of valproate has been successful in eliminating panic attacks with blood levels of the order of 77 mg/l being achieved (Roy-Burne et al, 1989).

Whilst TF eventually made good progress, more benefit may have been derived earlier if somewhat higher doses of the drugs prescribed had been tried before the treatment plan was changed.

With regard to gradual reduction of the daily dose of diazepam, it would have been advisable to have proceeded cautiously in view of the severity of his symptoms. The general recommendation is a reduction of 2 to 2.5 mg of diazepam per fortnight. An exacerbation of symptoms may be seen if the reduction is carried out more quickly than this.

4. Comment on the abrupt discontinuation of sertraline in this case.

Abrupt discontinuation of SSRIs can lead to a withdrawal syndrome characterised by electric shock sensations, dizziness, lethargy, paraesthesia, nausea, vivid dreams, irritability and lowered mood. This may complicate management if unrecognised. The incidence of such symptoms occurring upon the abrupt discontinuation of sertraline is said to be less than with some other members of this group (Coupland et al, 1996).

Key points

- The optimal treatment strategy for panic disorder is to suppress the symptoms of panic pharmacologically and then modify behaviour and cognition with cognitive behavioural therapy.

- Benzodiazepines offer relief in the short term.
- Tricyclics, MAOIs and SSRIs are all effective but may take four to six weeks to exert their full effect.
- Buspirone is ineffective in panic disorder.
- Propranolol and sodium valproate may be useful in some circumstances.

References

Aronson TA (1987) A naturalistic study of imipramine in panic disorder and agoraphobia, *Am J Psychiatry* **144:** 1014–19.

Bailly D (1996) The role of beta-adrenoreceptor blockers in the treatment of psychiatric disorders, *CNS Drugs* **5:** 110–23.

Ballenger JC, Wheadon DE, Steiner M et al (1998) Double-blind, fixed dose, placebo controlled study of paroxetine in the treatment of panic disorder, *Am J Psychiatry* **155:** 36–42.

Benjamin J, Levine J, Fox M et al (1995) Double blind, placebo-controlled, crossover trial of inositol treatment for panic disorder, *Am J Psychiatry* **152:** 1084–6.

Coupland NJ, Bell C, Potokar J (1996) Serotonin re-uptake inhibitor withdrawal, *J Psychopharmacol* **16:** 356–62.

Cowen PJ (1997) Pharmacotherapy for anxiety disorders: drugs available, *Adv Psychiatr Treat* **3:** 66–7.

Cross National Collaborative Panic Study (1992) Second phase investigations. Drug treatment of panic disorder, comparative efficacy of alprazolam, imipramine and placebo, *Br J Psychiatry* **160:** 191–202.

Gastfriend DR, Rosenbaum JF (1989) Adjunctive buspirone in benzodiazepine treatment for four patients with panic disorder, *Am J Psychiatry* **146:** 914–16.

Heninger GR, Charney DS (1988) Monoamine receptor systems and anxiety disorders. In: Winokur G, Coryell W, eds. *The Psychiatric Clinics of North America* (Philadelphia: W.B. Saunders).

Hoehn-Saric R, McLeod DR, Hipsley PA (1993) Efficacy of fluvoxamine in panic disorder, *J Clin Psychopharmacol* **13:** 321–6.

Klein DF (1964) Delineation of two drug-responsive anxiety syndromes, *Psychopharmacologia* **5:** 397–408.

Kostis JB (1990) CNS side effects of centrally acting antihypertensive agents: a prospective placebo-controlled study of sleep, mood state, and cognitive and sexual function in hypertensive males, *Psychopharmacology* **102:** 163.

Liebowitz MR (1989) Antidepressants in panic disorder, *Br J Psychiatry* **155:** (Suppl. 6), 46–52.

Modigh K, Westberg P, Eriksson E (1992) Superiority of clomipramine over imipramine in the treatment of panic disorder, *J Clin Psychopharmacol* **12:** 251–61.

Nutt D (1992) The role of benzodiazepine receptor in anxiety, *Psychiatry Pract* Summer, 5–7.

Oehrberg S, Christiansen PE, Behnke K (1995) Paroxetine in the treatment of panic disorder. A randomised, double-blind, placebo controlled study, *Br J Psychiatry* **167:** 374–9.

Priest RG (1990) Moclobemide and the reversible inhibitors of mono-amine oxidase antidepressants, *Acta Psychiatr Scand* **360:** 39–41.

Roy-Burne PP, Ward NG, Donnelly PJ (1989) Valproate in anxiety and withdrawal syndrome, *J Clin Psychiatry* **50:** (Suppl. 3), 44–8.

Sharp DM, Powers KG, Simpson RJ (1996) Fluvoxamine, placebo and cognitive behaviour therapy used alone and in combination in the treatment of panic disorder and agoraphobia, *J Anxiety Disord* **10:** 219–42.

Sheehan DV, Raj AB, Harnett–Sheehan K et al (1993) The relative efficacy of high-dose buspirone and alprazolam in the treatment of panic disorder: a double-blind placebo-controlled study, *Acta Psychiatr Scand* **88:** 1–11.

Suzman MM (1971) The use of beta-adrenergic blockade with propranolol in anxiety syndromes, *Postgrad Med* **47:** (Suppl), 104–7.

Wade AG, Lepola U, Koponen HJ et al (1997) The effect of citalopram in panic disorder, *Br J Psychiatry* **170:** 549–53.

Woodmen CL, Noyes R Jr (1994) Panic disorder: treatment with valproate, *J Clin Psychiatry* **55:** 134–6.

Antidepressant prophylaxis and discontinuation symptoms

Stephen Bazire

13

MF, a 48-year-old man, was readmitted to a psychiatric ward via casualty, bringing with him a box of venlafaxine 37.5 mg tablets, labelled 'take one twice a day'. He presented with a withdrawn and apathetic mood, appeared angry but there was no evidence of self-harm and neglect. The diagnosis was a relapse of depression. Although he had a number of social problems, his underlying problem was recurrent, poorly responsive depression, which was becoming chronic. He had been admitted to hospital for the treatment of depression five times in the previous eight years and had been prescribed antidepressants almost continuously since his index episode eight years ago. The treatment plan was to stabilise his mood with venlafaxine 150 mg/day and then discuss his long-term treatment.

MF attended one of the pharmacist-led medication education group sessions on the ward and it became evident that non-compliance with anti-

*depressants was likely to be a signifi-
cant factor in his case. One of the
reasons given by the patient for his
poor concordance with drug therapy
was his fear of becoming addicted to*
*antidepressants. This was reinforced
by his experiences of adverse experiences when stopping antidepressants
in the past, e.g. feeling as if he had
flu and 'sparks in the head'.*

Questions

1. How could you explain that antidepressants are not addictive?
2. Is MF likely to experience withdrawal or discontinuation effects when stopping antidepressants?
3. Is MF likely to relapse if he stops taking antidepressants again?

Answers

1. How could you explain that antidepressants are not addictive?

In a MORI poll carried out in 1991, 78% of the people interviewed agreed with the statement that 'antidepressants are addictive'. For a drug to be addictive, or produce dependence, it must have at least three of seven main features:

1. Tolerance to desired effect
2. Withdrawal symptoms
3. Use greater than needed
4. Inability to reduce the dose
5. Excessive time taken procuring the drug
6. Primacy of drug taking over other activities
7. Continued use despite understanding the adverse effects

One way of explaining to MF that an antidepressant is not addictive is to compare a variety of drugs and activities in terms of the first three mentioned characteristics and ask if the drug is used for an immediate effect or to help correct a suspected biological imbalance.

MF will be able to see that classic drugs of dependence produce craving, withdrawal symptoms and tolerance to their desired actions and are taken for

	Does the drug produce craving or desire?	Does the drug produce dependence?	Does the drug produce tolerance?	Does the drug correct a biological imbalance or is it taken for its immediate effect?
Alcohol	Yes	Yes e.g. 'DTs'	Yes	Effect
Caffeine	Yes	Yes e.g. headaches	Yes	Effect
Smoking	Yes	Yes	Yes	Effect
Amphetamines	Yes	Yes	Yes	Effect
Heroin etc	Yes	Yes e.g. 'cold turkey'	Yes	Effect
Gambling	Yes	Yes	Yes	Effect
Antidepressants	No	No	No	Correct imbalance
Hypnotics	Sometimes	Sometimes e.g. 'rebound' insomnia	Sometimes	Correct imbalance
Neuroleptics	No	No	No	Correct imbalance
Lithium	No	No, if done slowly over 4–12 weeks	No	Correct imbalance
Benzodiazepines	Sometimes but usually not with appropriate use	Sometimes	Sometimes	Correct imbalance

their immediate effect. Antidepressants do not cause craving and have no significant withdrawal symptoms; no tolerance to the therapeutic effects are seen and all help correct a presumed chemical imbalance in the brain.

2. Is MF likely to experience withdrawal or discontinuation effects when stopping antidepressants?

Withdrawal or discontinuation reactions have been reported for many anti-depressants. These withdrawal symptoms are not, however, indicative of dependence, as discussed above.

They are better described as 'discontinuation' effects or 'adjustment reactions'.

Discontinuation effects have a number of characteristics, e.g. they start within 1–2 days of stopping (longer for drugs with a longer half-life), resolve within 24 hours of restarting the drug and are common with longer courses or higher doses (Lejoyeux et al, 1996). At least eight weeks' treatment seems to be required before discontinuation symptoms occur, perhaps indicating that they are mediated through the longer term receptor changes induced by chronic antidepressant treatment (Lejoyeux et al, 1996). They can even occur with missed doses.

The main discontinuation symptoms with tricyclics include cholinergic rebound (e.g. headache, restlessness, diarrhoea, nausea and vomiting (Lieberman, 1981)), flu-like symptoms, lethargy, abdominal cramps, sleep disturbance and movement disorders. For SSRIs, the main symptoms are dizziness, vertigo/light-headedness, nausea, fatigue, headache, sensory disturbance, electric shocks in the head and limbs, insomnia, abdominal cramps, chills, increased dreaming, anxiety/agitation and volatility (Zajecka et al, 1997). Discontinuation symptoms usually persist for 7–14 days, although in some patients the duration may be many months (Gillespie et al, 1996).

Paroxetine has been associated with more withdrawal reports than the other SSRIs (Young et al, 1997), and this phenomenon may be because paroxetine inhibits its own metabolism and, as serum concentrations fall, less inhibition occurs and levels fall quicker, leading to a relatively rapid drop in plasma concentration (Preskorn, 1994). The CSM recommends slow tapering of

paroxetine if discontinuation symptoms occur; that is, stop, and if problems occur then restart and taper the dose downwards over 12 weeks, with either half-tablet doses or alternate day therapy. In a report of five cases of paroxetine withdrawal, however, even a four-week gradual discontinuation did not prevent significant symptoms of vertigo, light-headedness and gait instability, and so care is needed (Pacheco et al, 1996). The other SSRIs have fewer reported discontinuation effects. Fluoxetine has a long half-life and problems on discontinuation appear to be rare. Discontinuation symptoms are also probably less common with sertraline, fluvoxamine and citalopram than with paroxetine. Discontinuation effects on abrupt withdrawal from venlafaxine have included fatigue, headache, nausea, abdominal distention and congested sinuses (Farah and Lauer, 1996). A recent double-blind, placebo-controlled outpatient study showed that seven of the nine patients who discontinued sustained release venlafaxine reported the emergence of adverse reactions, compared with two of the nine patients who discontinued placebo (Fava et al, 1997).

It is thus quite possible that MF has had discontinuation effects, especially if he has stopped taking antidepressants abruptly in the past or has partially complied with short half-life antidepressants such as paroxetine. This will have re-inforced his view that antidepressants are addictive.

Treatment of discontinuation symptoms includes reinstatement at low dose and then tapering, use of an anticholinergic for symptomatic relief with tricyclics or just letting the symptoms resolve with reassurance (Garner et al, 1993).

3. Is MF likely to relapse if he stops taking antidepressants again?
It is known that 50–85% of people who suffer from one episode of major depression will go on to have further episodes, usually within two to three years if untreated, and that there is a high vulnerability in the early months after recovery.

There are a number of first-episode continuation treatment guidelines and recommendations. The American Psychiatric Association recommends at least 16–20 weeks' treatment at full dose after achievement of full remission, the WHO six months or more after recovery and the British Association for Psychopharmacology Consensus Committee at least four

months after the patient is apparently well (BAP Consensus Committee, 1993). Subsequent episodes usually require longer treatment. Continuation doses should be the same as or close to the therapeutic dose (Frank et al, 1993).

Risk factors for relapse include recurrent dysthymia, concurrent non-affective psychiatric illness, chronic medical disorder and a history of relapses. Increasing severity of subsequent episodes is predicted by serious suicide attempts, psychotic features or severe functional impairment (Kupfer et al, 1992). MF is thus at high risk of relapse after recovery and is a long-term risk if untreated.

There are many studies showing prevention of relapse by tricyclics (e.g. Frank et al, 1993), fluoxetine (Montgomery et al, 1988) and sertraline (Doogan and Caillard, 1992). Probably the best study is by Frank et al (1990), a three-year study with a two-year follow-up (Kupfer et al, 1992). One hundred and twenty-eight patients with recurrent depression (third or more episode of depression) who had responded to imipramine plus interpersonal therapy were evaluated. All were symptom free at the start of the trial.

After three years, around 75% of those receiving imipramine remained well compared with less than 15% receiving placebo. The relapsers in the active treatment group were mainly non-compliers. Those patients remaining well on imipramine at the end of the original three-year study period were randomised to continue with active treatment or to receive placebo. After a further two-years, 82% of those randomised to receive active treatment remained well, compared with 33% of those who received placebo.

The message for MF is thus clear. Antidepressants are effective, they are not addictive and will prevent relapse if he takes them long-term.

Key points

- 78% of the general public agree with the statement 'antidepressants are addictive'.
- Antidepressants do not cause craving and have no significant withdrawal symptoms; no tolerance to their therapeutic effect is seen, and they all help to correct a presumed 'chemical imbalance' in the brain.
- Discontinuation symptoms usually occur one to two days after anti-depressants are stopped, and last for 7–14 days if untreated.
- At least eight weeks' treatment with an antidepressant seems to be required before a significant risk of discontinuation symptoms occurs.
- Shorter half-life drugs are associated with a higher incidence of discontinuation symptoms than longer half-life drugs.
- In a cohort of patients who had suffered from at least three episodes of depression, 75% of those randomised to receive imipramine for three years remained well, compared with less than 15% of those randomised to receive placebo. This benefit continued for at least a further two years.

References

British Association for Psychopharmacology Consensus Committee (1993) Guidelines for treating depressive illness with antidepressants, *J Psychopharmacol* **7:** 19–23.

Doogan DP, Caillard V (1992) Sertraline in the prevention of depression, *Br J Psychiatry* **160:** 217–22.

Farah A, Lauer TE (1996) Possible venlafaxine withdrawal syndrome, *Am J Psychiatry* **153:** 576.

Fava M, Mulroy R, Alpert J et al (1997) Emergence of adverse events following discontinuation of treatment with extended-release venlafaxine, *Am J Psychiatry* **154:** 1760–2.

Frank E, Kupfer DJ, Perel JM et al (1990) Three year outcome for maintenance therapies in recurrent depression, *Arch Gen Psychiatry* **47:** 1093–9.

Frank E, Kupfer DJ, Perel JM et al (1993) Comparison of full-dose versus half-dose pharmacotherapy in the maintenance treatment of recurrent depression, *J Affect Disord* **27:** 139–45.

Garner EM, Kelly MW, Thompson DF (1993) Tricyclic antidepressant withdrawal syndrome, *Ann Pharmacother* **27:** 1068–72.

Gillespie C, Wildgust HJ, Haddad P (1996) SSRIs and withdrawal syndrome. Abstract G2389 X, *World Congress of Psychiatry,* Madrid.

Kupfer DJ, Frank E, Perel JM et al (1992) Five year outcome for maintenance therapies in recurrent depression, *Arch Gen Psychiatry* **49:** 769–73.

Lejoyeux M, Ades J, Mourad I et al (1996) Antidepressant withdrawal syndrome. Recognition, prevention and management, *CNS Drugs* **5:** 278–92.

Lieberman J (1981) Cholinergic rebound in neuroleptic withdrawal syndromes, *Psychosomatics* **22:** 253–4.

Montgomery SA, Dufour H, Brion S et al (1988) The prophylactic efficacy of fluoxetine in unipolar depression, *Br J Psychiatry* **153:** (Suppl. 3), 69–76.

Pacheco L, Malo P, Aragues E et al (1996) More cases of paroxetine withdrawal syndromes, *Br J Psychiatry* **169:** 384.

Preskorn S (1994) Targeted pharmacotherapy in depression management: comparative pharmacokinetics of fluoxetine, paroxetine and sertraline, *Int Clin Psychopharmacol* **9:** (Suppl. 3), 13–19.

Young AH, Currie A, Ashton CH (1997) Antidepressant withdrawal syndrome, *Br J Psychiatry* **170:** 288.

Zajecka J, Tracy KA, Mitchell S (1997) Discontinuation symptoms after treatment with serotonin reuptake inhibitors: a literature review, *J Clin Psychiatry* **58:** 291–7.

Antidepressant therapeutic drug monitoring and drug interactions

Carol Paton

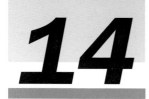

JB, a 36-year-old woman, was brought to psychiatric outpatients by her concerned sister, two weeks before her routine appointment. Her mood was subjectively and objectively low, with marked anhedonia. She exhibited marked psychomotor retardation and had difficulty concentrating during the interview. JB reported poor sleep with both initial insomnia and early morning wakening. Appetite was poor with weight loss of around a stone in the last month, and she appeared clinically dehydrated. She admitted to thoughts of death, wishing that she would die in her sleep rather than having any active suicide plans.

JB had a nine-year history of recurrent unipolar depression with several admissions to hospital, the last one being a three-month admission one year ago. She was treated with amitriptyline 200 mg at night, which she had taken since, and remained relatively well until one month ago.

JB was admitted to hospital, re-hydrated, and her permission was sought for ECT. Both the patient and her family were strongly opposed to this option. The consultant decided to respect their wishes as long as there was no further deterioration and meanwhile requested blood to be taken for an amitriptyline serum level.

The amitriptyline serum level was reported as 180 ng/ml. As this patient had failed to respond to more conventional augmentation strategies, such as lithium, in the past, the decision was taken to add fluvoxamine 50 mg to the amitriptyline.

Five days later the patient was complaining that she felt worse than ever, with a very dry mouth and blurred vision. She had marked postural drop (120/70 to 80/40) and a tachycardia (p120 bpm). She was not clinically dehydrated.

Questions

1. Why was an amitriptyline plasma level requested and how can it help the management of this case?
2. Explain the side-effects experienced after the addition of fluvoxamine.
3. Which other commonly prescribed drugs interact with SSRIs?
4. Do any of the other new antidepressants inhibit hepatic metabolising enzymes to a degree likely to cause drug interactions?

Answers

1. Why was an amitriptyline plasma level requested and how can it help the management of this case?

The patient in this case had been doing well until a month ago on a relatively high dose of amitriptyline. The plasma level may have been requested to check compliance or whether the plasma amitriptyline concentration was in the 'therapeutic range' from both an efficacy and a potential toxicity perspective.

In order for plasma levels (therapeutic drug monitoring: TDM) to be useful for any drug, certain criteria should apply (Evans et al, 1986):

1. There should be an accepted therapeutic range that has been established through clinical trials.
2. There should be a wide variation in individual drug handling.
3. Plasma levels should relate directly to clinical and adverse effects.
4. There should be a narrow therapeutic index with significant consequences from treatment failure or toxicity.

Studies which have aimed to determine a 'therapeutic range' for amitriptyline have not produced entirely consistent results, although a target range of 100–200 ng/ml for amitriptyline and 50–150 ng/ml for nortriptyline are generally accepted (Taylor and Duncan, 1995). This inconsistency is not surprising when it is considered that around a third of depressed patients are placebo-responders, that some will experience a natural remission in their illness, and that not every patient with a plasma level in the 'therapeutic range' will respond (only two-thirds can be expected to). For the first two groups, plasma levels are irrelevant to outcome, and in the third group it is not usually possible to identify responders and non-responders before a drug trial. In addition, it is often assumed that only tertiary and secondary amines are active

antidepressants, although it is known that their various hydroxylated metabolites penetrate the CNS and are active. For amitriptyline and nortriptyline, the 10-hydroxy-metabolites can occur at levels greater than those of the parent compound (Bertilsson et al, 1979).

Although some authors agree that there is a wide variation in individual drug handling (Taylor and Duncan, 1995), others are more sceptical. Work done at the Geoffrey Knight Unit for resistant affective disorders demonstrated that, when blood was taken at a standard time (12 hours post-dose) at steady state (at least a week after a change in dose), and the effects of co-medication were accounted for (concurrent hepatic enzyme inducers such as carbamazepine or inhibitors such as thioridazine), there was little inter-patient variability between dose and plasma level for dothiepin (Hodgkiss, 1993). The effects of co-medication can be significant: in this cohort of patients, three out of four who received carbamazepine in combination with dothiepin 300–550 mg/day had plasma dothiepin plus major metabolites levels of less than 200 ng/ml.

Hodgkiss (1993) noted that 'treatment refractory' patients were unlikely to respond to plasma levels of dothiepin plus major metabolites of less than 200 ng/ml, while serious side-effects (severe tremor, falls, tachycardia) were more likely above 500 ng/ml.

Concurrent physical pathology can also significantly alter tricylic plasma levels: for example, raised plasma alpha$_1$-glyco-protein can lead to vastly increased plasma tricyclic levels (albeit temporarily) due to increased protein binding (Glassman et al, 1985).

The prediction that tricyclic plasma levels were likely to grow in usefulness (Glassman et al, 1985) has only been partially realised.

In conclusion, amitriptyline plasma levels can be useful:

1. When non-compliance is suspected,
2. To ensure adequate plasma levels in refractory depression,
3. To avoid serious adverse drug reactions,
4. To monitor the effects of co-medication.

In the case of JB, the plasma level could exclude relapse due to non-compliance and indicate whether dosage adjustment might be appropriate.

2. Explain the side-effects experienced after the addition of fluvoxamine.

The selective serotonin re-uptake inhibitors (SSRIs) are potent inhibitors of several of the cytochrome liver enzymes, although all have different patterns of inhibition (Nemeroff et al, 1996). The cytochrome liver enzymes detoxify many substances that are foreign to the body including drugs and environmental toxins. The long-term consequences of inhibition of some or all of these enzymes are unknown (Lane et al, 1995). Amitriptyline is partly metabolised via cytochrome P4501A2, and fluvoxamine is a potent inhibitor of this enzyme. Plasma amitriptyline levels are likely to rise dramatically and pronounced side-effects appear, as in this case. The other SSRIs are significantly less potent at inhibiting P4501A2, but all inhibit to varying degrees P4502C, P4502D6 and P4503A4 (Nemeroff et al, 1996; Taylor and Lader, 1996).

Cytochrome P4502D6 exhibits genetic polymorphism, with 5–10% of the Caucasian population lacking this enzyme because of an autosomal recessive transmitted defect in its expression. P4502D6 is required for the metabolism of the secondary amines nortriptyline and desipramine (Nemeroff et al, 1996), and is inhibited by paroxetine, fluoxetine and sertraline. Case reports have been published which describe fluoxetine 20 mg increasing nortriptyline plasma levels by 375% (Vaughan, 1988), and sertraline 50 mg increasing plasma desipramine levels by 150% (Barros and Asnis, 1993). It is important to note that enzyme inhibition is dose dependent and that the higher doses of sertraline used clinically are likely to have a more pronounced effect than that described above.

P4502C also exhibits polymorphism with 3–5% of the Caucasian population lacking the enzyme. P4502C is required for the metabolism of tertiary amines such as amitriptyline, clomipramine and imipramine, and is inhibited by fluvoxamine, fluoxetine and sertraline.

P4503A4 constitutes 60% of the metabolising capacity of the liver. Amitriptyline and imipramine are metabolised by P4503A4 and this enzyme is inhibited by fluvoxamine, nefazodone, norfluoxetine, sertraline and paroxetine (Nemeroff et al, 1996), although the degree of inhibition varies substantially and is arguable in some cases (fluvoxamine, sertraline and paroxetine).

Our knowledge of the exact roles of the various cytochrome enzymes and

the individual patterns and consequences of inhibition by various drugs is in its infancy and much remains to be understood. It is, however, clear that SSRIs and tricyclics should not be prescribed together unless tricyclic plasma levels are measured (Taylor, 1995). The need for caution extends to the change-over period when switching from a tricyclic to an SSRI (when the tricyclic dose should be reduced substantially in the days before change-over), or fluoxetine to a tricyclic (when a lower initial dose of tricyclic should be used, possibly several weeks, to compensate for the long half-life of fluoxetine and its metabolite).

3. Which other commonly prescribed drugs interact with SSRIs?
Cytochrome P4501A2 at least partly metabolises theophylline, caffeine, clozapine, haloperidol, some tricyclics including amitriptyline and olanzapine. The metabolism of all of these drugs is potently inhibited by fluvoxamine. Fluoxetine has also been reported to inhibit significantly the metabolism of clozapine although the exact mechanism is unclear (Taylor, 1997).

Fluvoxamine, fluoxetine and sertraline, through inhibition of P4502C, raise plasma concentrations of diazepam, clomipramine, amitriptyline, warfarin (increased clotting time and minor haematuria reported), phenytoin (up to 300% increases) and tolbutamide.

Fluoxetine, sertraline and paroxetine, through inhibition of P4502D6, can raise plasma levels of haloperidol, fluphenazine, risperidone, sertindole, various beta-blockers and codeine.

Nefazodone and fluoxetine, and possibly sertraline, paroxetine and fluvoxamine, through inhibition of P4503A4, can lead to higher plasma levels of benzodiazepines, terfenadine, astemizole, carbamazepine, calcium channel blockers, erythromycin, steroids, codeine and quinidine. These interactions are reviewed in detail by Nemeroff et al (1996) and Taylor and Lader (1996). Citalopram appears to have fewer effects on hepatic cytochrome enzymes and may be the SSRI of choice when a significant interaction can be anticipated in a patient who is already receiving a drug with a narrow therapeutic range such as phenytoin or warfarin.

4. Do any of the other new antidepressants inhibit hepatic metabolising enzymes to a degree likely to cause drug interactions?
Yes.

Nefazodone is a potent inhibitor of CYP3A4 and a weak inhibitor of CYP2D6 (Nemeroff et al, 1996). Moclobemide inhibits CYP2C, and to a lesser extent, CYP1A2 and CYP2D6 (Gram et al, 1995). Venlafaxine inhibits CYP2D6, although this effect is less potent than that shown by the SSRIs (Holliday and Benfield, 1995). Mirtazapine is a weak inhibitor of CYP1A2, CYP2D6 and CYP3A4 and clinically significant drug interactions seem unlikely (Stimmel et al, 1997), while reboxetine would seem to be devoid of activity on any of the important drug-metabolising enzymes (Dostert et al, 1997).

Key points

* Tricyclic plasma levels can be useful when non-compliance is suspected, to ensure adequate plasma levels in refractory depression, to avoid serious side-effects and to monitor the effects of co-medication on tricyclic metabolism.
* Most SSRIs are potent inhibitors of hepatic cytochrome enzymes, each demonstrating a different pattern of inhibition.
* SSRIs (except citalopram) potently inhibit the metabolism of tricyclics, and co-prescription is contraindicated

unless tricyclic plasma levels are monitored.

- SSRIs inhibit the metabolism of many commonly prescribed drugs including some with a narrow therapeutic index such as phenytoin and warfarin. These interactions can be predicted for each SSRI from their individual patterns of cytochrome enzyme inhibition.
- All other new antidepressants, with the exception of reboxetine, inhibit hepatic cytochrome enzymes to varying degrees.

References

Barros J, Asnis G (1993) An interaction of sertraline and desipramine, *Am J Psychiatry* **150:** 1751. Correction (1994) **151:** 300.

Bertilsson L, Mellstrom B, Sjoqvist F (1979) Pronounced inhibition of noradrenaline uptake by 10-hydroxy-metabolites of nortriptyline, *Life Sci* **25:** 1285–92.

Dostert P, Benedetti MS, Poggesi I (1997) Review of the pharmacokinetics and metabolism of reboxetine, a selective noradrenaline reuptake inhibitor, *Eur Neuropsychopharmacol* **7:** S23–S25.

Evans WE, Schentag JJ, Jusco WJ (1986) *Applied Pharmacokinetics: Principles of Therapeutic Drug Monitoring.* (Vancouver: Applied Therapeutics).

Glassman AH, Schilkraut JJ, Orsulak PJ et al (1985) Tricyclic antidepressant blood level measurements and clinical outcome: an APA task force report, *Am J Psychiatry* **142:** 155–62.

Gram LF, Guentert TW, Grange S et al (1995) Moclobemide, a substrate of CYP2C19 and an inhibitor of CYP2C19, CYP2D6 and CYP1A2: a panel study, *Clin Pharmacol Ther* **57:** 670–7.

Hodgkiss A (1993) *Tricyclic plasma levels revisited.* United Medical & Dental Schools (Guy's Campus) Ego, *Bull Div Psychiatry* Autumn, 56–63.

Holliday S, Benfield P (1995) Venlafaxine: a review of its pharmacology and therapeutic potential in depression, *Drugs* **49:** 280–94.

Lane R, Baldwin D, Preskorn S (1995) The SSRIs: advantages, disadvantages and differences, *J Psychopharmacol* **9:** 163–78.

Nemeroff CB, DeVane CL, Pollock BG (1996) Newer antidepressants and the cytochrome P450 system, *Am J Psychiatry* **153:** 311–20.

Stimmel GL, Dopheide JA, Stahl SM (1997) Mirtazapine: an antidepressant with noradrenergic and specific serotonergic effects, *Pharmacotherapy* **17:** 10–21.

Taylor D (1995) Selective serotonin reuptake

inhibitors and tricyclic antidepressants in combination: interactions and therapeutic uses, *Br J Psychiatry* **167:** 575–80.

Taylor D (1997) Pharmacokinetic interactions involving clozapine, *Br J Psychiatry* **171:** 109–12.

Taylor D, Duncan D (1995) Plasma levels of tricyclics and related antidepressants: are they necessary or useful? *Psychiatr Bull* **19:** 548–50.

Taylor D, Lader M (1996) Cytochromes and psychotropic drug interactions, *Br J Psychiatry* **168:** 529–32.

Vaughan DA (1988) Interaction of fluoxetine with tricyclic antidepressants, *Am J Psychiatry* **145:** 1478.

Refractory depression

Railton Scott

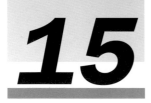

TR, a 45-year-old man, was admitted to an acute psychiatric ward following an outpatient appointment. He appeared anxious and agitated. TR's mental state examination revealed diurnal variation of mood with early morning wakening, decreased appetite with associated weight loss and anhedonia. On direct questioning, TR admitted to feeling suicidal at times, although he denied any specific plans to kill himself. There were no psychotic features.

TR was first seen by the psychiatric services two years ago, following the death of his mother. He was treated with fluoxetine at that time and has taken it intermittently since. TR is unmarried and lives alone in rented accommodation. He worked for many years as an antique furniture restorer, but was retired on health grounds one year ago. TR is in debt to credit card companies and to his sister. He smokes 30 cigarettes daily and is a social drinker. TR has a six-year history of diet-controlled NIDDM and has chronic hip pain due to a motorcycle accident 15 years ago. Drugs on admission were fluoxetine 20 mg daily (taken for 10 weeks), temazepam 20 mg at night and indomethacin SR 75 mg at night.

Routine blood tests (U&Es, LFTs, TFTs, FBC) fasting blood sugar and glycosy-lated haemoglobin were normal.

On admission, TR's prescription was changed to paroxetine 20 mg/day, and increased to 50 mg/day over the next eight weeks with little change in his mental state.

Questions

1. Discuss the appropriateness of TR's past and current antidepressant treatment.
2. Describe and explain a typical pharmacological treatment algorithm for refractory depression.
3. Are there any other points that should be considered in this case?
4. What is the prognosis in patients with treatment-refractory depression?

Answers

1. Discuss the appropriateness of TR's past and current antidepressant treatment.

Fluoxetine, a selective serotonin re-uptake inhibitor (SSRI), is an effective and well-established treatment for depression. Therapeutic efficacy is thought to be achieved by increased concentrations of 5-hydroxytryptamine (5HT) at the postsynaptic receptor site (Rickles and Schweizer, 1990).

However, there are at least two reasons why fluoxetine may not have been the antidepressant of choice in TR. Firstly, fluoxetine, as with other SSRIs, can have an alerting effect, which may account for an exacerbation of the anxiety/agitation suffered by TR (Wernicke et al, 1987). Approximately 15% of patients on fluoxetine complain of these effects. Secondly, TR has a diagnosis of NIDDM and fluoxetine may not be appropriate in this condition (Salmon, 1995).

Adverse effects of fluoxetine such as tremor, sweating, nausea and anxiety may mimic a hypoglycaemic attack. In addition, fluoxetine may increase peripheral and hepatic insulin action. This may induce hypoglycaemia on starting treatment and hyperglycaemia when the drug is stopped. TR, however, had normal fasting glucose and glycosylated haemoglobin levels.

Of more concern in this case is that TR had been taking fluoxetine 20 mg daily for 10 weeks with minimal response. Changing to paroxetine, which has essentially the same mode of action, is illogical. An antidepressant from a different class would be a more appropriate second step. It should be noted that caution should be shown when changing from fluoxetine to a tricyclic, as fluoxetine is a potent inhibitor of several hepatic metabolising enzymes and can significantly raise tricyclic serum levels (Taylor and Lader, 1996). The long half-life of fluoxetine can thus complicate management in the changeover period.

2. Describe and explain a typical pharmacological treatment algorithm for refractory depression.

TR has had a therapeutic dose of fluoxetine for 10 weeks, followed by paroxetine for eight weeks. He was an inpatient for the second treatment trial, and whilst this is by no means a guarantee of compliance, compliance was not in doubt in this case.

At this stage TR should be prescribed a tricyclic antidepressant in place of the SSRI. Features of his depression include a poor sleep pattern and agitation, making a sedating tricyclic such as amitriptyline an appropriate choice. Plasma levels of tricyclics and their active metabolites can be measured. This can be used to confirm treatment adherence and to facilitate dosage titration and optimisation (Hodgkiss et al, 1995). The dosage required for most tricyclics is unlikely to be less than 150 mg/day and may be considerably higher.

Although there is no accepted definition for treatment-refractory depression, most psychiatrists would accept that patients who have reached this point with minimal response could be described as having treatment-refractory illness. This would be in agreement with Remick (1989), who suggested 'unsuccessful treatment with at least two antidepressants and/or a course of ECT' as a working definition. Recent work has indicated that repeated drug trials may lessen subsequent antidepressant effectiveness. It has been estimated that the response rate for subsequent antidepressant therapy is reduced by as much as 20% for each treatment failure (Amsterdam and Maislin, 1994). Lack of prompt treatment for clinical depression is known to be a risk factor for the development of treatment-refractory illness (Smith, 1995). It follows that depressive illness should be treated vigorously. Treatment options are briefly described below.

Lithium, which is widely used as a mood-stabilising agent in bipolar depression, has also been successfully used to augment antidepressant therapy in treatment-resistant depression (Pope et al, 1988). In some cases, response to the addition of lithium was rapid (de Montigny et al, 1981), whilst others (Thase et al, 1989) reported that the response to the addition of lithium was more gradual and occurred over a period of weeks rather than days. Recent work (Cornelius et al, 1995) has demonstrated that lithium augmentation could also be of benefit when augmenting SSRI therapy. In addition, this study highlighted the need for adequate plasma levels of lithium (at least 0.4 mmol/l). If lithium is to be used as an augmentation agent, then plasma levels must be optimised and monitored. Therapeutic levels of lithium should be maintained for a minimum period of six weeks.

A further augmentation strategy is the use of tri-iodothyronine (T3) to potentiate thyroid function. Indeed, use of T3 supplementation was first described over three decades ago (Prange et al, 1969). Hypothyroidism is well known to exacerbate or even cause depression and all patients with treatment-refractory depression should have thorough thyroid function testing. Subsequent research (Targum et al, 1984) has shown that patients with subclinical hypothyroidism responded to supplementation with thyroxine (T4) whereas euthyroid patients showed a substantially higher response when treated with T3 (Joffe and Singer, 1991). Euthyroid patients who are non-responsive to optimised antidepressant treatment should have a four-week trial of T3 at a daily dose of 25–50 µg, if they have no contraindications to its use. Higher doses for longer periods may result in hypothyroidism on subsequent discontinuation.

Electroconvulsive therapy (ECT) remains a treatment option at any time, should TR be at risk of self-injury or suicide or endanger his physical health by not eating or drinking. A detailed discussion of ECT is beyond the scope of this book, but numerous reviews exist (e.g. Potter and Rudorfer, 1993).

If TR has still not responded to treatment after the above interventions, several other treatment options are worth considering. It must be emphasised that efficacy data for all of these options are very limited.

Some success has been claimed for pindolol, a β-adrenoceptor and presynaptic $5HT_{1A}$ antagonist. The $5HT_{1A}$ presynaptic autoreceptor, when stimulated by serotonin, reduces the amount of serotonin released into the synpatic cleft. Antagonists at this receptor would therefore be expected to block this negative feedback mechanism (which may be activated by antidepressants), thus allowing greater amounts of serotonin to activate post-synaptic receptors and, theoretically, relieve depression. One study which randomised patients to receive placebo or pindolol 7.5 mg/day in addition to fluoxetine (Perez et al, 1997) found that the number of days required to reach a sustained response was lower in the pindolol group (19 versus 29 days) and the overall response rate was

higher (69 versus 48%). These findings were not replicated by Berman et al (1997). Other studies have been conducted, but the effect of pindolol is still not clear.

Venlafaxine may also be an option. In an open trial of 84 patients with treatment-resistant depression, one-third were considered to have responded after 12 weeks' treatment, and half of this group sustained their response for a further three months (Nierenberg et al, 1994). It should be noted that there was no placebo or active comparator drug arm in this study, and that the mean dose of venlafaxine was 245 mg, rather higher than that used in normal clinical practice.

Success has also been claimed for some antidepressant combinations. In all cases, these combinations should only be prescribed with caution, systematically, and by a team experienced in their use. The risk/benefit ratio should be carefully evaluated and discussed fully and frankly with the patient (Amsterdam and Hornig-Rohan, 1996). One option is to use a combination of an SSRI and a tricyclic, usually nortriptyline (Seth et al, 1992). If such combinations are used, it is advisable to monitor tricyclic serum levels and

ECG. Fluoxetine in particular may elevate tricyclic levels through inhibition of the hepatic-metabolising enzyme CPY2D6 (Taylor and Lader, 1996). Moreover, the combination of a tricyclic and an SSRI is thought by some not to have proven efficacy (Taylor, 1995).

A further option is the combination of a tricyclic and a MAOI (Marley and Wozniak, 1983). The combination of clomipramine and tranylcypromine is absolutely contraindicated, as fatalities have been reported. Other combinations may also be highly dangerous.

Another combination worth mentioning is clomipramine, L-tryptophan (available on a named patient basis) and lithium (Hale et al, 1987).

If the above fail, sleep deprivation, bright light therapy, or psychosurgery may be options worth considering (Singh, 1995).

3. Are there any other points that should be considered in this case?

All patients with treatment-refractory depression should have their diagnosis reviewed to exclude physical causes or any other factors that may complicate management. TR has suffered the loss of his mother and his work, may be socially isolated and is in debt. In addition, he has NIDDM and suffers from chronic pain. All of these factors can predispose to the development of treatment-refractory depression (Smith, 1995). Intervention in any of these areas may be helpful.

TR is also prescribed indomethacin, which is known to cause depression (Indocid Data Sheet, 1996), albeit rarely.

4. What is the prognosis in patients with treatment-refractory depression?

A National Institute of Mental Health (NIMH) study (Winokur et al, 1993) found that 50% of patients who had a diagnosis of treatment-resistant depression recovered within three years. The need for ongoing active management of these patients is emphasised.

Key points

- Patients who do not respond to an adequate dose and adequate duration of one antidepressant should be given a trial of a second antidepressant from a different class.
- Tricyclic plasma levels can be useful in optimising therapy.

- Lithium (serum levels > 0.4 mmol/l) or tri-iodothyronine (25–50 mg/day) can be useful adjuncts.
- Other options include pindolol, venlafaxine, combinations of SSRIs and tricyclics, tricyclics and MAOIs, and clomipramine, L-tryptophan and lithium. These options should be used with care and under expert advice.
- Sleep deprivation, bright light therapy and psychosurgery may be options worth exploring.
- All patients with treatment-refractory depression should have their case thoroughly reviewed to exclude organic or drug-induced causes. Psychosocial interventions may be possible and fruitful.
- Fifty per cent of patients diagnosed as having treatment-refractory depression recover within three years.

References

Amsterdam JD, Hornig-Rohan M (1996) Treatment algorithms in treatment-resistant depression, *Psychiatr Clin North Am* **19:** 371–86.

Amsterdam JD, Maislin G (1994) Fluoxetine efficacy in treatment-resistant depression, *Prog Neuropsychopharmacol Biol Psychiatry* **18:** 243–61.

Berman RM, Darnell AM, Miller HL et al (1997) Effect of pindolol in hastening response to fluoxetine in the treatment of major depression: double blind, placebo controlled trial, *Am J Psychiatry* **154:** 37–43.

Cornelius LE, Katona MT, Abou-Saleh DA et al (1995) Placebo controlled trial of lithium augmentation of fluoxetine and lofepramine, *Br J Psychiatry* **166:** 80–6.

De Montigny C, Grunberg F, Meyer A et al (1981) Lithium induces rapid relief of depression in TCA drug non-responders, *Br J Psychiatry* **138:** 252–6.

Hale AS, Procter AW, Bridges PK (1987) Clomipramine, tryptophan and lithium in combination for resistant endogenous depression: seven case studies, *Br J Psychiatry* **151:** 213–7.

Hodgkiss AD, McCarthey PT, Sulke AN et al (1995) High dose tertiary amine tricyclic antidepressants in the treatment of refractory depression: the central role of plasma concentration estimations, *Hum Psychpharmacol* **10:** 407–15.

Indocid Data Sheet. *Data Sheet Compendium 1996–7.* (London: Datapharm Publications).

Joffe RT, Singer W (1991) Thyroid hormone potentiation of antidepressants. In: Amsterdam JD, ed. *Refractory Depression.* (New York: Raven Press), 185–90.

Marley E, Wozniak KM (1983) Clinical and

experimental aspects of interaction between amine oxidase inhibitors and amine re-uptake inhibition, *Psychol Med* **13:** 735–49.

Nierenberg AA, Feighner JP, Rudlph R et al (1994) Venlafaxine for treatment-resistant unipolar depression, *J Clin Psychopharmacol* **14:** 419–23.

Perez V, Gilaberte I, Faries D (1997) Randomised, double-blind, placebo-controlled trial of pindolol in combination with fluoxetine antidepressant treatment, *Lancet* **349:** 1594–7.

Pope HG, McElroy SL, Nixon RA (1988) Possible synergism between fluoxetine and lithium in refractory depression, *Am J Psychiatry* **145:** 10.

Potter WZ, Rudorfer MV (1993) Electroconvulsive therapy: a modern medical procedure, *N Eng J Med* **328:** 882–3.

Prange AJ, Wilson IC, Rabon AM et al (1969) Enhancement of imipramine anti-depressant activity by thyroid hormone, *Am J Psychiatry* **126:** 39–51.

Remick RA (1989) Treatment resistant depression, *Psychiatr J Univ Ottawa* **14:** 394–6.

Rickels K, Schweizer E (1990) Clinical overview of serotonin reuptake inhibitors, *J Clin Psychiatry* **51:** (B Suppl.), 9–12.

Salmon G (1995) Use of fluoxetine in patients with diabetes mellitus, *Psychiatr Bull* **19:** 553–4.

Seth R, Jennings AL, Bindman J (1992) Combination treatment with noradrenaline and serotonin reuptake in resistant depression, *Br J Psychiatry* **161:** 562–5.

Singh SP (1995) Treatment resistant depression: causes and consequences, *Psychiatr Bull* **19:** 680–5.

Smith AJ (1995) Treatment resistant depression: causes and consequences, *Psychiatr Bull* **19:** 676–80.

Targum SD, Greenberg RD, Harmen RL et al (1984) The TRH test and thyroid hormone in refractory depression [letter], *Am J Psychiatry* **141:** 463.

Taylor D (1995) Selective serotonin reuptake inhibitors and tricyclic antidepressants in combination. Interactions and therapeutic uses, *Br J Psych* **167:** 575–80.

Taylor D, Lader M (1996) Cytochromes and psychotropic drug interactions, *Br J Psychiatry* **168:** 529–32.

Thase ME, Kupfer DJ, Frank E et al (1989) Treatment of imipramine-resistant recurrent depression: an open, clinical trial of lithium augmentation, *J Clin Psychiatry* **50:** 413–17.

Wernicke JF, Dunlop SR, Dornseif BE et al (1987) Fixed dose fluoxetine therapy for depression, *Psychopharmacol Bull* **23:** 164–8.

Winokur G, Coryell W, Keller M et al (1993) A prospective follow-up of patients with bipolar and primary unipolar affective disorder, *Arch Gen Psychiatry* **50:** 457–65.

Treatment of depression in people with epilepsy

Denise Duncan

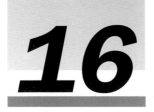

SC, a 25-year-old Caucasian woman who has a ten-year history of complex partial seizures with a temporal lobe focus and secondary generalised seizures, was seen in casualty 12 hours after a flurry of secondary generalised tonic clonic seizures. She presented with acute suicidal thoughts and severe depression. Symptoms included anhedonia, loss of appetite, sleep disturbance, loss of sexual desire and suicidal ideation. Her GP had diagnosed depression one month previously and had prescribed dothiepin. SC was unemployed, precluded from driving because of her epilepsy and had recently broken up with her long-term boyfriend. Her medication at presentation was:

> Dothiepin 225 mg nocte
>
> Carbamazepine 200 mg nocte   Plasma level = 4 mg/l
>
> Primidone 250 mg nocte   (range: 4–12)

Questions

1. What are the contributing factors for depression seen in SC and what other contributing factors are there in people with epilepsy?
2. What factors may have contributed to her recent flurry of seizures?
3. What are the important factors to consider in the treatment of depression in people with epilepsy?

Answers

1. What are the contributing factors for depression seen in SC and what other contributing factors are there in people with epilepsy?

The causes of depression in epilepsy are complex and may be related to the treatment of SC's epilepsy, to psychosocial factors, to an underlying pathology causing both the seizures and the depression or may be unrelated to epilepsy. Some of the drugs used in the treatment of epilepsy can cause depression, either directly or indirectly. For example, phenobarbitone and primidone (which is metabolised to phenobarbitone) directly cause depression. Depression resulting from antiepileptic drug (AED)-induced folate deficiency or from stigma resulting from the appearance and social embarrassment of gingival hyperplasia caused by phenytoin are examples of indirect effects.

Psychosocial factors include stigma and public perceptions, restrictions on driving, difficulties in gaining employment and self-esteem issues. Structural, developmental or genetic abnormalities may be responsible for both seizures and depression but, of course, SC may have simply developed a primary depressive illness (McConnell and Duncan, 1998).

Factors which may have been responsible for SC's depressive illness include stigma, unemployment, being prevented from driving, her recent relationship break-up, primidone therapy, epilepsy with a temporal lobe focus and loss of seizure control.

2. What factors may have contributed to her recent flurry of seizures?

Factors which could have contributed include:

- A subtherapeutic carbamazepine level. Even though her plasma level of 4 mg/l is within the reference range for carbamazepine, this is not controlling her seizures. The dose should be titrated upwards to maximise control. Note also that once-daily administration of carbamazepine, particularly in a patient receiving an enzyme-inducing drug such as primidone, is highly unlikely to lead to therapeutic blood levels over a 24-hour period.
- SC's recently prescribed dothiepin. Tricyclic antidepressants (TCAs) can lower the seizure threshold, especially if they are started at too high a dose and increased too quickly. SC's dothiepin plasma level should be measured.
- Stress, such as the recent break-up of her relationship.
- Primidone inducing carbamazepine's metabolism and thus lowering its plasma level (if primidone had recently been added to SC's carbamazepine therapy).
- Depression, possibly increasing seizure frequency. A causal relationship is not certain.
- Lack of adherence to her prescribed anticonvulsants. Although there is no direct evidence in this case, missed medication is one of the common causes of seizure exacerbation and should always be considered.

3. What are the important factors to consider in the treatment of depression in people with epilepsy?

Before an antidepressant is prescribed to someone with epilepsy it is essential to determine whether the depression has a temporal relationship with the seizures (peri-ictal) or whether it has occurred independently of the seizures (inter-ictal). In peri-ictal depression it is important to optimise AED therapy and not to give an antidepressant that could further lower the seizure threshold and thus contribute towards further depressive episodes. In inter-ictal depression an antidepressant should be chosen that is less likely to lower the seizure threshold, or to interact with any prescribed medication, or cause unacceptable adverse effects.

Seizures are an infrequent but important adverse effect of most, if not all, available antidepressants. Risk factors for antidepressants causing seizures include epilepsy or a previous history of seizures, head injury or loss of consciousness; known EEG abnormalities; a history of substance abuse or withdrawal from alcohol or anxiolytics;

dementia; a recent or rapid dose escalation of the antidepressant; and high plasma levels of the drug or its metabolites. (For a full review see McConnell and Duncan (1998).) Some antidepressants may also be more likely to induce seizures in a given individual. As there are no comparative studies examining antidepressants in epilepsy with respect to seizures, it is necessary to use animal, clinical trial, EEG and overdose data, case reports, prescription event monitoring and reports from the Committee on Safety of Medicines (CSM) to evaluate the seizure potential of a given antidepressant.

If all of the above are considered, it appears that the selective serotonin re-uptake inhibitors (SSRIs) and moclobemide are less likely to lower the seizure threshold than TCAs (McConnell and Duncan, 1998). Of the TCAs, it appears that dothiepin may be one of the more epileptogenic antidepressants. In one overdose study, dothiepin was much more likely to cause seizures than were other TCAs (Buckley et al, 1994), although this was probably at least partly because those patients who had taken dothiepin had consumed much larger doses than those patients who had taken other TCAs. Figures from

the United States indicate that dothiepin has a higher incidence of seizures (0.89%) than other TCAs (0.5%) (de Jonghe and Swinkles, 1992). Clomipramine also appears to be one of the more epileptogenic antidepressants. In one study a seizure incidence of 1.04% was found (Waalinder and Feighner, 1992), although seizure rates have been quoted as being 0.48-2.1% with the highest risk occurring on doses above 300 mg/day (Stimmel and Dopheide, 1996). Dothiepin and clomipramine should be avoided in people with epilepsy. If a TCA is to be given, doxepin may be the drug of choice. In a study in which doxepin was given to people with epilepsy, seizure frequency increased in only two of 19 patients, whereas 15 patients had a decrease in seizure frequency and in two it was unchanged (Ojemann et al, 1983).

If an SSRI is to be chosen, there is some evidence that fluoxetine and sertraline may be less epileptogenic and paroxetine and fluvoxamine more epileptogenic (McConnell and Duncan, 1998). Overdose data for trazodone suggest that it may also be a drug that is less likely to lower the seizure threshold (Wedin et al, 1986) and could be a useful antidepressant if sedation is required.

Once it has been decided which antidepressants are safest with respect to seizure threshold, potential drug interactions need to be considered. As carbamazepine is metabolised by cytochrome p4503A4 (CYP3A4), any drug that is metabolised by, or is an inhibitor or inducer of CYP3A4 could potentially interact with carbamazepine. For instance, norfluoxetine (the principal metabolite of fluoxetine) is a potent inhibitor of CYP3A4, as is nefazodone. Fluoxetine and nefazodone would therefore be expected to increase carbamazepine plasma levels. Indeed, fluoxetine has been shown to increase carbamazepine plasma levels by up to 60%, resulting in carbamazepine toxicity (Pearson, 1990). These drugs should therefore generally be avoided in patients taking carbamazepine.

Sertraline is thought to be less likely to raise carbamazepine plasma levels. Nevertheless, there has been one report in which carbamazepine plasma levels were increased by 80% within four weeks of sertraline 100 mg being started (Joblin and Ghose, 1994). Fluvoxamine has also been reported to

increase carbamazepine plasma levels (Fritze et al, 1991).

Another AED with a narrow therapeutic index is phenytoin. Phenytoin is metabolised by cytochrome CYP2C9 and CYP2C19 and thus fluoxetine, a known inhibitor of CYP2C19, could increase phenytoin plasma levels. This has been borne out in practice (Woods et al, 1994; Jalil, 1992). Serum levels need to be monitored closely. Sertraline (Ciraulo et al, 1995) has also been reported to raise plasma levels, although not to a clinically significant degree and there is an unpublished study of paroxetine increasing phenytoin levels (cited by McConnell and Duncan, 1998). Although fluoxetine is the drug most likely to interact with both carbamazepine and phenytoin (and nefazodone with carbamazepine), plasma levels of these two AEDs should be monitored closely after the addition of any new antidepressant, since pharmacokinetic interactions can rarely be discounted.

Conversely, it is possible that the AED enzyme inducers (carbamazepine, phenytoin, phenobarbitone and primidone) could lower antidepressant plasma levels, and sodium valproate, an enzyme inhibitor, could increase antidepressant plasma levels.

Both valproate and, to a lesser extent carbamazepine, can cause weight gain and many of the AEDs can cause drowsiness. It may be preferable to choose an antidepressant that is less likely to cause these adverse effects, namely an SSRI.

If we consider all of the above, the antidepressants of choice in people with epilepsy are fluoxetine (if there are no interacting drugs, or if careful monitoring is available), sertraline and moclobemide. MAOIs may also be suitable but should, in theory, not be given with carbamazepine. Trazodone is an option if sedation is required. If a TCA is required, doxepin is probably the drug of choice.

Key points

- Underlying physical pathology, psychosocial factors and anticonvulsant drugs may all contribute to the development of depression in people with epilepsy.
- It is important to determine whether the depression is peri-ictal or inter-ictal before embarking on a treatment regimen.
- Peri-ictal depression should be dealt with by optimising anticonvulsant cover.

- Inter-ictal depression necessitates the use of antidepressants.
- SSRIs, MAOIs and moclobemide are less epileptogenic than tricyclics.
- Potential drug interactions between anticonvulsants and SSRIs should be considered.

References

Buckley NA, Dawson AH, Whyte IM et al (1994) Greater toxicity in overdose of dothiepin than of other tricyclic antidepressants, *Lancet* **343:** 159–62.

Ciraulo DA, Shader RI, Greenblatt DJ et al (1995) *Drug Interactions in Psychiatry.* Baltimore: Williams & Wilkins.

De Jonghe F, Swinkles JA (1992) The safety of antidepressants, *Drugs* **43:** (Suppl. 2), 40–7.

Fritze J, Unsorg B, Lanczik M (1991) Interaction between carbamazepine and fluvoxamine, *Acta Psychiatr Scand* **84:** 583–4.

Jalil P (1992) Toxic reaction following the combined administration of fluoxetine and phenytoin: two case reports, *J Neurol Neurosurg Psychiatry* **55:** 412–13.

Joblin M, Ghose K (1994) Possible interaction of sertraline with carbamazepine, *NZ Med J* **107:** 43.

McConnell HW, Duncan D (1998) The treatment of psychiatric comorbidity in epilepsy. In: McConnell HW, Snyder PJ, eds. *Psychiatric Comorbidity in Epilepsy: Basic Mechanisms, Diagnosis and Treatment.* (Washington DC: American Psychiatric Press) 245–361.

Ojemann LM, Friel PN, Trejo WL et al (1983) Effect of doxepin on seizure frequency in depressed epileptic patients, *Neurology* **33:** 646–8.

Pearson HJ (1990) Interaction of fluoxetine with carbamazepine, *J Clin Psychiatry* **51:** 126.

Stimmel GL, Dopheide JA (1996) Psychotropic drug-induced reductions in seizure threshold: incidence and consequences, *CNS Drugs* **5:** 37–50.

Waalinder J, Feighner JP (1992) Novel selective serotonin reuptake inhibitors, part 1, *J Clin Psychiatry* **53:** 107–12.

Wedin GP, Oderda GM, Klein-Schwartz W et al (1986) Relative toxicity of cyclic antidepressants, *Ann Emergency Med* **15:** 797–804.

Woods DJ, Coulter DM, Pillans P (1994) Interaction of phenytoin and fluoxetine, *NZ Med J* **107:** 970.

Antidepressant-induced switching in bipolar affective disorder

Shameem Mir

17

CM, a 27-year-old Caucasian woman, was arrested by the police after refusing to pay for an expensive meal in the local Holiday Inn Hotel. CM was running around the restaurant bare-footed, brandishing a scarf above her head. She was very agitated and exhibited pressure of speech and flight of ideas. She was well dressed in expensive flamboyant clothes, was wearing heavy, bright make-up and her hair was somewhat dishevelled. CM was taken to hospital by the police on a Section 136.

CM's first psychiatric admission was nine years ago with a diagnosis of a hypomanic episode which responded to antipsychotic treatment. Her second admission was a year later with the same diagnosis. At this time lithium was prescribed. CM had been stable on lithium for the first two years but then started to suffer from major depressive episodes. Over the last six years she has had five admissions; three for major depression and two for hypomania, both of which occurred around

6–8 weeks after starting antidepressant therapy (amitriptyline and then fluoxetine). During CM's last admission (12 weeks ago) she was prescribed venlafaxine, the dose of which had been cautiously increased over two months to 75 mg twice a day. CM had been prescribed this dose for four weeks prior to her current presentation.

CM had no significant medical history. Her mother had a diagnosis of bipolar affective disorder; her mental state had remained stable on lithium therapy for the past 20 years. CM was admitted to hospital. Her drug regime on admission was lithium carbonate 800 mg at night and venlafaxine 75 mg twice a day.

A physical examination and routine blood tests were unremarkable. CM's 12-hour lithium level on admission was 0.8 mmol/l and a urine drug screen proved negative.

The working diagnosis was hypomania, probably induced by antidepressants.

Questions

1. What is antidepressant-induced switching and what is its prevalence?
2. What is the optimum treatment for CM?

Answers

1. What is antidepressant-induced switching and what is its prevalence?

Switching is the induction by antidepressants of mania or hypomania in patients with unipolar or bipolar disorder. It can also indicate an antidepressant-induced increase in cycle rate.

The major problem in trying to establish the frequency of antidepressant-induced mania is that any 'switch' could be part of the natural course of the illness. It is generally accepted that all antidepressants have the potential to induce mania or accelerated cycling, but there are few data comparing the incidence or severity of these effects between the different classes of antidepressants. One of the reasons for such scant data is that clinical trials involving antidepressant drugs often exclude patients with a history of bipolar disorder. In addition, large clinical trials of antidepressants in combination with mood stabilisers have not been conducted since the early 1980s.

The studies conducted to date have many shortfalls: early studies did not separate bipolar and unipolar patients; few were placebo controlled; phases of illness differed between acute and continuation therapy; some groups contained a higher proportion of women; and those studies conducted in tertiary referral centres may have included 'difficult to treat' patients who may be more prone to switching. With these caveats in mind, the following studies are of note.

A switch rate of 41% has been reported in bipolar patients who are medication free (Lewis and Winokur, 1982). In a review of 15 placebo-controlled studies that included over 1200 patients (Rouillon et al, 1992) the switch rate in unipolar patients randomised to receive tricyclics was 1–5%, compared wirh 0–9% of those randomised to receive placebo. Of the 158 patients diagnosed as having bipolar illness, the switch rate was reported as 23% with placebo,

21% with lithium alone, 28% with lithium in combination with a tricyclic and 51% with a tricyclic alone. These results would indicate that half of the switch rate in this patient group may be due to the natural course of the illness, and the other half due to treatment with tricyclics, or perhaps simply the occurrence of depression.

In a retrospective study of patients with refractory bipolar illness, Altshuler et al (1995) concluded that mania was likely to have been induced by antidepressants in one-third of cases and cycle acceleration in a quarter. These observations were supported by a later naturalistic, prospective study (cited by Post et al, 1997).

Altshuler et al (1995) also found that antidepressant-induced cycle acceleration was associated with younger age at first treatment and more likely to occur in women (later supported by Simpson and Liebowitz, 1996). They also found bipolar patients to be particularly at risk. These findings contradict those of an earlier study by Kupfer et al (1988), who found no difference in the incidence of antidepressant-induced switching between unipolar and bipolar groups. Altshuler et al (1995) also described the course of illness in a treatment-refractory cohort of patients. Such patients are likely to have an illness pattern in which mania follows depression (Faedda et al, 1991) and this should be considered when their results are interpreted.

Peet (1994) compared the incidence of switch into mania using pooled data from trials of selective serotonin reuptake inhibitors (SSRIs), tricyclic antidepressants (TCAs) and placebo. For those with unipolar illness the switch rate for SSRIs, TCAs and placebo were 0.72%, 0.52% and 0.21%, respectively. For those with a bipolar illness, the switch rates were 3.7%, 11.2% and 4.2%. From this, Peet concluded that SSRIs were the antidepressants of choice in those with a history of bipolar disorder. Vesely et al (1997), however, advised caution in the use of SSRIs and reported six cases of SSRI-induced mania (four of which were on above the maximum recommended BNF dose of antidepressant).

This variation in switch rates lends support to the theory that it is the antidepressant and not the depression which is largely responsible for switching.

Case reports of antidepressant withdrawal precipitating hypomania have also been published (e.g. Nelson et al, 1983; Gupta and Narang, 1986). Such reports are infrequent and difficult to interpret. The withdrawal of lithium may precipitate a manic episode (Schou, 1993). Carbamazepine withdrawal has also been implicated (Scull and Trimble, 1995).

2. What is the optimum treatment for CM?
CM has a diagnosis of bipolar affective disorder. She has had five hypomanic episodes (three thought to be antidepressant-induced) and three episodes of depression over the previous nine years. CM has been taking lithium carbonate for the past eight years. Although lithium is a widely accepted treatment for the prophylaxis of bipolar disorder, it does not appear to have been effective in this patient. In a recent review, Moncrieff (1997) questioned the efficacy of lithium in the treatment of acute mania, unipolar and bipolar disorders. Cookson (1997) argued that lithium is effective in some patients for prophylactic therapy in bipolar disorder and that it is important to establish whether the patient is a 'lithium responder' first. It may be worth considering an alternative mood stabiliser such as carbamazepine or sodium valproate or the addition of one of these drugs to her current regimen.

Carbamazepine has both mood-stabilis-ing (Disalver et al, 1996) and perhaps antidepressant effects (Post et al, 1986; Stuppaeck et al, 1994). Sodium val-proate has been shown to be beneficial for treating both mania and rapid cycling (Schaff et al, 1993), and Swann et al (1997) have reported superiority to lithium in treating symptoms of depression during mania.

Consideration also needs to be given to CM's antidepressant therapy, without which she is susceptible to depressive episodes but with which she appears to become hypomanic. The data comparing the incidence of antidepres-sant-induced switching with different classes of antidepressants is still arguably inconclusive. Indeed, this patient has experienced switching with a tricyclic, serotonin reuptake inhibitor and now venlafaxine. CM should ideally be maintained on mood-stabilising drugs, alone or in combination. Antidepressants should be reserved for severe episodes of depression. Verapamil, a calcium channel blocker, has mood-stabilising effects (Giannini et al, 1984) and case reports of its success in preventing antidepressant-induced mania in otherwise refractory patients have been published (Gitlin and Weiss, 1984).

Key points

- Switching is the induction by antidepressants of mania or hypomania in patients with unipo-lar or bipolar disorder.
- Approximately 50% of bipolar patients, if treated with a tricyclic alone during a depressive episode, will switch into hypomania.
- Lithium has a protective effect.
- There are few comparative data between different antidepressants, although SSRIs may be associated with a lower risk than tricyclics.
- Bipolar patients should ideally be maintained with mood-stabilising drugs either alone or in combina-tion.
- Antidepressants should generally be reserved for severe depressive episodes.

References

Altshuler LL, Post RM, Leverich GS et al (1995) Antidepressant-induced mania and cycle acceleration: a controversy revisited, *Am J Psychiatry* **152:** 1130–8.

Cookson J (1997) Lithium: balancing risks and benefits, *Br J Psychiatry* **171:** 120–4.

Disalver SC, Swann SC, Chen Y et al (1996) Treatment of bipolar depression with carbamazepine: results of an open study, *Biol Psychiarty* **40:** 935–7.

Faedda GL, Baldessarini RJ, Tohen M et al (1991) Episode sequence in bipolar disorder and response to lithium treatment, *Am J Psychiatry* **148:** 1237–9.

Giannini AJ, Houser WL, Loiselle RH et al (1984) Antimanic effects of verapamil, *Am J Psychiatry* **141:** 1602–3.

Gitlin MJ, Weiss J (1984) Verapamil as maintenance treatment in bipolar illness: a case report, *J Clin Psychopharmacol* **4:** 341–3.

Gupta R, Narang RI (1986) Mania induced by gradual withdrawal from long-term treatment with imipramine, *Am J Psychiatry* **143:** 260.

Kupfer DJ, Carpenter LL, Frank E (1988) Possible role of antidepressants in precipitating mania and hypomania in recurrent depression, *Am J Psychiatry* **145:** 804–8.

Lewis JL, Winokur G (1982) The induction of mania: a natural history study with controls, *Arch Gen Psychiatry* **39:** 303–6.

Moncrieff J (1997) Lithium: evidence reconsidered, *Br J Psychiatry* **171:** 113–19.

Nelson JC, Schottenfeld RS, Conrad CD (1983) Hypomania after desipramine withdrawal, *Am J Psychiatry* **140:** 624–5.

Peet M (1994) Induction of mania with selective serotonin re-uptake inhibitors and tricyclic antidepressants, *Br J Psychiatry* **164:** 549–50.

Post RM, KIrk DD, Leverich GS et al (1997) Drug-induced switching in bipolar disorder: epidemiology and therapeutic indications, *CNS Drugs* **8:** 352–65.

Post RM, Uhde TW, Roy-Byrne PP et al (1986) Antidepressant effects of carbamazepine, *Am J Psychiatry* **143:** 29–34.

Rouillon F, Lejoyeux M, Filteau MJ (1992) Unwanted effects of long term treatment. In: Montgomery SA, Rouillon F, eds. *Long Term Treatment of Depression.* (New York: John Wiley & Sons).

Schaff MR, Fawcett J, Zajecka JM (1993) Divalproex sodium in the treatment of refractory affective disorders, *J Clin Psychiatry* **54:** 381–5.

Schou M (1993) Is there a lithium withdrawal syndrome? An examination of the evidence, *Br J Psychiatry* **163:** 514–18.

Scull DA, Trimble MR (1995) Mania precipitated by carbamazepine withdrawal, *Br J Psychiatry* **167:** 698.

Simpson HB, Liebowitz MR (1996) Antidepressant-induced cycle acceleration in bipolar affective disorder, *Am J Psychiatry* **153:** 1239.

Stuppaeck CH, Barnas C, Schwitzer J et al (1994) Carbamazepine in the prophylaxis of major depression: a 5-year follow-up, *J Clin Psychiatry* **55:** 146–50.

Swann AC, Bowden CL, Morris D et al (1997) Depression during mania: treatment response to lithium or divalproex, *Arch Gen Psychiatry* **54:** 37–42.

Vesely C, Fischer P, Goessler R et al (1997) Mania associated with selective serotonin reuptake inhibitors, (Letter). *J Clin Psychiatry* **58:** 88.

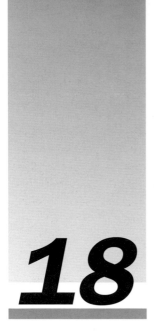

Mania

Peter Pratt

MP, a 54-year-old lady was admitted to an acute psychiatric ward after being found outside her house earlier in the day, dressed in her night attire. A member of the public had complained that she had become verbally aggressive when she refused to join her in saving the world.

It was difficult to obtain a full history from MP as her speech was rapid and made little sense. She often made reference to being God and her need to save the world. MP would often break into song, 'Oh what a beautiful morning', in the middle of a sentence.

MP lived on her own and had no recent contact with her family. She had one daughter from a previous marriage which had ended 15 years previously. MP had not worked since her father's newsagent business closed in the 1970s.

MP had records of two previous admissions, two and five years ago. Her records indicate she had received lithium, carbamazepine, haloperidol, droperidol and chlorpromazine at various times during these admissions often in combination. She had not recently been prescribed any medication and a urine screen confirmed she had not been taking any illicit drugs. There appeared to be no obvious precipitant to this episode.

On the ward MP was sexually disinhibited, asking other patients to have sex with her and produce God's children. On occasions she became verbally aggressive, particularly when other patients asked her to leave them alone. Mental state examination revealed several grandiose delusions. MP was diagnosed as having an episode of mania.

Questions

1. Discuss the pharmacological treatment options for an episode of mania.
2. Formulate a drug treatment plan for MP.

Answers

1. Discuss the pharmacological treatment options for an episode of mania.

Any physical basis for MP's symptoms should be identified and appropriately treated. Such causes would include cerebral disorders, infections and drug or alcohol misuse. Many prescribed drugs have been reported to induce mania, particularly antidepressants and steroids.

The choice of treatment for an episode of mania includes lithium, antipsychotics and carbamazepine, and combi-

nation strategies involving these drugs may be employed. Benzodiazepines and electroconvulsive therapy (ECT) also have a role. Other treatment options include other anticonvulsants, calcium channel blockers (Dubovsky et al, 1986; 1995) and beta blockers. If episodes recur, then longer-term prophylactic treatment should be considered.

Moncrieff (1997) and Cookson (1997) have debated the relative pros and cons of treatment with lithium. These two reviews contained few common references and could be criticised as being biased, albeit opposing views, where the authors selectively searched the literature in order to locate references which were in line with their opinions. Despite the confusion caused by the two opposing views presented in these reviews and the paucity of good quality randomised controlled trials, lithium is still considered by many clinicians to be first line prophylactic treatment of bipolar disorder. Moreover, premature termination of lithium prophylaxis leads to a high relapse rate (Suppes et al, 1991). This should be discussed with the patient before prescribing lithium and a minimum duration of treatment of at least three years agreed.

In the acute phase, prompt treatment is essential. The patient may be at physical risk through exhaustion and their actions may lead to financial disaster for themselves and their family. Reckless behaviour may result in loss of employment or criminal conviction. Loss of life or injury to the patient or others may occur if the patient continues with potentially dangerous activities such as driving. Increased sexual activity may lead to pregnancy, sexually transmitted disease and in some cases may make it difficult for the patient to

return to their friends or family. Suicidal thoughts are uncommon in pure mania but may occur in more than 50% of cases when symptoms of both mania and depression occur nearly every day (a mixed mood state) (Dilsaver et al, 1994).

Debate continues over which agent, or combination is the treatment of choice for an episode of mania. Moncrieff (1997) points out the lack of clear cut benefit for lithium as demonstrated by randomised clinical trials. Others claim that some studies do show evidence for the benefit of lithium in the milder forms of mania (Chou, 1991; Cookson, 1997; Dali, 1997). Nevertheless, an increased interest in using lithium (or alternatives) has been fuelled by concerns over the potential side effects of antipsychotic drug treatment.

To be an effective antimanic agent, lithium needs to be given in sufficient dosage to produce 12-hour lithium levels of around 1.0–1.2 mmol/l. Even then, response may be delayed for up to 10 days. The risk of lithium toxicity when treating an episode of mania is significant. There can be great variability in fluid intake and physical exertion, and physical monitoring may be difficult.

Within the UK at least, it is common practice to use alternatives to lithium in the management of severe mania and those with psychotic symptoms (Peet and Pratt, 1993). Antipsychotics are considered to be effective in the treatment of mania, but again randomised clinical trials are few. The small numbers of studies account for the observation that different authors give completely different views. Moncrieff (1997) feels the majority of studies demonstrate the superiority of antipsychotics over lithium, whereas Bowden (1996) suggests that from randomised comparisons, antipsychotics are consistently shown to be less effective than lithium.

The impression of most clinicians is that antipsychotics are effective in mania and that they appear to have a more rapid effect than lithium (Chou, 1991). Chlorpromazine is the antipsychotic that has been most frequently studied but trials involving other antipsychotics appear to show similar benefits, leading Chou (1991) to conclude that there is little difference in antimanic response between individual antipsychotics, particularly in controlling hyperactivity. Nevertheless, the use of flupenthixol may be unwise, in view of the manufacturer's SPC (summary of product charac-

teristics). This includes advice that this drug is not suitable for agitated or excited patients.

In routine clinical practice haloperidol is often cited as the antipsychotic of choice. Others suggest the additional sedative effects of chlorpromazine or droperidol render them superior, particularly in the first few days of treatment. Where medication must be given parentally, zuclopenthixol acetate, formulated as a longer acting injection (Clopixol Acuphase) may offer practical advantages when repeated IM injections might otherwise be necessary.

There is an increasing trend towards using lower doses of antipsychotics in clinical practice, as there is limited, but convincing evidence, that there is a potent argument for using the smallest dose possible for the shortest period of time. Increasing the dose of haloperidol above 10 mg per day in the management of mania confers no additional benefit (Rifkin et al, 1994). If additional sedation is required, adjunctive treatment with a benzodiazepine would appear less hazardous than increasing the doses of antipsychotic. The only therapeutic benefit from higher doses of antipsychotics would be as an attempt to exploit any secondary sedative effect of the antipsychotics. This additional sedative action is often misinterpreted as antipsychotic action.

There are case reports which suggest clozapine and risperidone may be effective in mania, but in general the use of atypical antipsychotics has not been fully evaluated. This is unfortunate, as it has been suggested that patients with bipolar illness may be at a higher risk of tardive dyskinesia and other extrapyramidal side effects than those with schizophrenia.

Evidence in support of carbamazepine in the treatment of mania is limited and the drug is not licensed for this purpose in the UK. Various reviews, including those incorporating open studies and case reports suggest a response rate of around 60% in mania (Chou, 1991; Elphick, 1989). Sub groups of manic patients likely to respond to carbamazepine have not been clearly identified. Empirically there appears to be support for using carbamazepine in those patients refractory to lithium, typically those with rapid cycling bipolar disorder (see case on Rapid Cycling).

Response to carbamazepine is likely to occur from around five days to one month after initiation of treatment. Carbamazepine dosage should be titrated slowly from 200 mg once or twice daily (at least every 5 days in the early part of treatment) until either the patient responds, or is unable to tolerate further increases. Carbamazepine plasma levels do not appear to correlate with response, but may also help to predict toxicity. Inadequate dose could explain an apparent lack of response, if steady state plasma levels of less than 7 mg/l are achieved (Taylor and Duncan, 1997). Carbamazepine should only be considered for the treatment of an episode of mania if other treatment options are either ineffective or impracticable.

Some limited evidence exists to support the use of the higher potency benzodiazepines, clonazepam and lorazepam as anti manic agents in their own right (Santos and Morton, 1989; Bottai et al, 1995). A case can be made for benzodiazepines both enhancing the antipsychotics effects of neuroleptics, and having an independent antipsychotic effect of their own (Wolkowitz et al, 1991).

In routine clinical practice the major role for benzodiazepines appears to be in combination with antipsychotics or lithium. The aim is to produce a rapid calming effect without resorting to large doses of antipsychotics, or to produce rapid control of psychomotor agitation until the antimanic effects of the other treatment has become apparent. Lorazepam and diazepam are available as parenteral as well as oral forms. Diazepam should not be given intramuscularly as absorption is - unpredictable. Treatment with benzodiazepines should be considered a short-term strategy as tolerance and dependence are likely to occur with longer-term treatment.

Concern has been expressed that the combination of lithium and haloperidol may produce irreversible brain damage. However, as long as excessive doses of both are avoided and fluid intake maintained, antipsychotics can normally be considered to be safe in combination with lithium. The risk of extrapyramidal reactions or neuroleptic malignant syndrome may be increased when lithium and antipsychotics are co-prescribed which is why some clinicians favour combinations of antipsychotics with carbamazepine or sodium valproate.

There is limited evidence to suggest that valproate may be more effective as a prophylaxis against manic episodes than depressive episodes. The use of valproate and other anticonvulsants is covered in the Rapid Cycling case.

2. Formulate a drug treatment plan for MP. Pharmacological treatment is important. MP is clearly at risk of being exploited or harmed by others. She may assault other patients and appears to have little insight into her condition.

As far as is possible, MP should be assessed to ensure she is physically well, with no apparent contraindications to drug treatment. Possible precipitating causes such as drugs of abuse, or prescribed drugs such as steroids, should be excluded. MP's previous episodes may provide useful information on the effect of medication and the time course for response.

Target symptoms should be documented.

As MP's mania presents with psychotic symptoms, initial treatment should be with an antipsychotic. A benzodiazepine should be used to provide additional sedation. Treatment should start with haloperidol 5 mg twice daily and lorazepam 2 mg twice daily. Other neuroleptics such as droperidol could be considered as alternatives. Written and verbal explanation of the treatment should be given to MP.

If MP does not accept oral medication, consideration should be given to administering medication against her wishes under the Mental Health Act. Clopixol Acuphase may be used instead of repeated IM doses of haloperidol.

If symptoms of disinhibition have not improved within seven days consideration should be given to increasing the dose of benzodiazepine and antipsychotic. MP's delusional belief that she is God and needs to save the world may take several weeks to respond. It is very unlikely, however, that doses higher than 15 mg of haloperidol per day will increase the speed of MP's response.

In recovery, the duration of sleep may be a good indicator for judging the rate of benzodiazepine reduction. Haloperidol should not be discontinued prematurely.

As this is MP's third episode of mania within five years, consideration should be given to prescribing prophylactic medication. Lithium is the treatment of choice. Time must be spent in helping MP understand the implications of long term treatment with lithium. Lithium should not be prescribed unless MP is in agreement with the plan that it should be taken for several years (preferably at least three years).

Key points

- Antipsychotics and benzodiazepines in combination are the drugs most frequently prescribed to treat an episode of mania.
- Haloperidol is probably the antipsychotic of choice, although the sedative effects of chlorpromazine and droperidol are considered by some to be useful.
- The non-specific sedative effects of antipsychotics should not be confused with their antipsychotic action.
- Benzodiazepines usefully augment the efficacy of antipsychotics.
- Lithium, carbamazepine, other anticonvulsants, calcium channel blockers and ECT are other options.
- The risk of manic relapse after discontinuation of lithium is high. This should be considered before prescribing lithium to treat an episode of mania.

References

Bottai T, Hue B, Hillaire-Buys D et al (1995) Clonzaepam in acute mania: time blind evaluation of clinical response and concentrations in plasma, *J Affect Disord* **36:** 21–7.

Bowden CL (1996) Dosing strategies and time course of response to antimanic drugs, *J Clin Psychiat* **57:**(Suppl. 13), 4–9.

Chou JC-Y (1991) Recent advances in treatment of acute mania, *J Clin Psychopharm* **11:** 3–21.

Cookson J (1997) Lithium: balancing the risks and benefits, *Br J Psych* **171:** 120–4.

Dali I (1997) Mania, *Lancet* **349:** 1157–60.

Dilsaver SC, Chen YW, Swann AC et al (1994) Suicidality in patients with pure and depressive mania, *Am J Psych* **15:** 1312–15.

Dubovsky SL, Franks RD, Allen S (1986) Calcium antagonists in mania: a double blind study of verapamil, *Psych Res* **18:** 309–20.

Dubovsky SL, Buzan RD (1995) The role of calcium channel blockers in the treatment of psychiatric disorders, *CNS Drugs* **4:** 47–54.

Elphick M (1989) Clinical issues in the use of carbamazepine in psychiatry: a review, *Psych Med* **19:** 591–604.

Moncrieff J (1997) Lithium: evidence reconsidered, *Br J Psych* **171:** 113–19.

Peet M, Pratt JP (1993) Lithium current status in psychiatric disorders, *Drugs* **4:** 7–17.

Rifkin A, Doddi S, Karajgi B et al (1994) Dosage of haloperidol for mania, *Br J Psych* **165:** 113–16.

Santos AB, Morton WA (1989) Use of benzodiazepines to improve management of manic agitation, *Hosp and Comm Psych* **40:** 1069–71.

Suppes T, Baldessanni RJ, Faedda GL (1991) Risk of recurrence following discontinuation of lithium treatment in bipolar disorder, *Arch Gen Psych* **48:** 1082–8.

Taylor D, Duncan D (1997) Doses of carbamazepine and valproate in bipolar affective disorder, *Psych Bull* **21:** 221–3.

Wolkowitz OM, Pickar D (1991) Benzodiazepines in the treatment of schizophrenia: a review and reappraisal, *Am J Psych* **148:** 714–26.

Lithium prophylaxis, withdrawal and use in pregnancy

Stephen Bazire

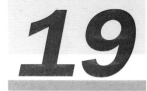

NH, an intelligent, 35-year-old woman with a stable bipolar mood disorder had been prescribed lithium 600 mg at night for six years following two major hypomanic episodes. Since then, she had been stable for four years. NH had one depressive episode five years ago, during which she made an attempt to take her own life. NH has been married for three years and has been functioning well. She attended a routine outpatient appointment, where she announced that she had stopped taking her lithium three days ago as she would like to start a family. (Her GP had advised her that lithium was teratogenic.)

Questions

1. What are the main advantages for NH of continuing to take lithium?
2. What problems might be expected if lithium is stopped abruptly as with NH?
3. What problems might be anticipated when lithium is taken during pregnancy?

Answers

1. What are the main advantages for NH of continuing to take lithium?

Lithium is widely used for the treatment and prophylaxis of bipolar affective disorder. There are nine major placebo-controlled trials of lithium as prophylaxis of bipolar disorder and although most have methodological flaws (e.g. most used a lithium-withdrawal control group), their findings are considered of great importance (Goodwin, 1995). Prophylactic use of lithium can, with appropriate care and monitoring, be both effective and safe. Lithium must be taken regularly and monitored correctly, and the risks and benefits of ongoing treatment must be regularly reviewed, with consideration to the clinical circumstances of each individual case.

The prophylactic efficacy of lithium is probably maintained over at least ten years (Berghofer et al, 1996). Firm data are also accumulating that long-term lithium treatment markedly reduces the excess mortality of people with recurrent affective disorders (Muller-Oerlinghausen et al, 1996), most probably by reducing the suicide rate (Gershon and Soares, 1997). Conversely, discontinuation of lithium prophylaxis has been shown to be associated with elevated rates of psychiatric hospitalisation and use of emergency services (Johnson and McFarland, 1996).

Refractoriness to lithium despite adequate lithium levels, induced by lithium discontinuation in previously lithium-responsive patients, has been reported many times (e.g. Bauer, 1994; Maj et al, 1995). There is, however, some dispute about this, since a well-designed study that followed 86 patients over two lithium maintenance treatment periods (mean four years each) was unable to demonstrate this phenomenon (Tondo et al, 1997). In this study it is of note that no difference in response rates was seen between the first and second treatment periods, irrespective of the gap between treatment periods or the rate of discontinuation of lithium after the first treatment period. This is particularly interesting, as it is an established fact that patients with bipolar disorder tend to have more frequent episodes as they get older.

Thus, the prevention of relapse, suicide risk protection and possible prevention of future refractoriness are suggested major advantages of continuing lithium for someone like NH, who has an established bipolar illness.

2. What problems might be expected if lithium is stopped abruptly as with NH?
Early relapse in bipolar illness following lithium discontinuation is well accepted. The risk of recurrence (predominantly of mania) in bipolar

disorder may be up to 28 times higher in the first three months after stopping lithium than it is for those patients who continue to take lithium (Suppes et al, 1991). This recurrence rate may even exceed that of untreated bipolar illness.

Two papers have illustrated the danger of abrupt discontinuation. The first (Baldessarini et al, 1996) studied 161 people who had been taking lithium for an average of four years and who wanted to stop. One group stopped abruptly (over 1–14 days) and the second stopped gradually (over 15–30 days). Both groups were followed for 3.5 years. The relapse rates are shown in Table 1.

Over the first year, those who stopped lithium abruptly were three times as likely to relapse compared with those who stopped gradually, but the rate of relapse was the same in both groups

Table 1
Relapse rates after lithium withdrawal

	Gradual withdrawal (15–30 days)	Abrupt withdrawal (1–14 days)
Bipolar I	78% had relapsed at 3 years	100% had relapsed within 3 years
Bipolar II	50% had relapsed at 3.5 years	100% had relapsed within 3.5 years

after one year. Overall, those who stopped lithium gradually were substantially more likely to remain in remission than if they had stopped lithium abruptly. The average time to relapse was six months for the 'abrupt stoppers', and 15 months for the 'gradual stoppers'. The second study (Baldessarini et al, 1997) followed 78 people with bipolar disorder over two years. Again, one group stopped lithium abruptly (over 1–14 days) and another group stopped gradually (over 15–30 days). The 'time to relapse' was nearly six times as long for the gradual stoppers (14 months) compared with abrupt stoppers (2.5 months). Around 95% of the abrupt stoppers relapsed within two years, whereas only 69% of the gradual stoppers had relapsed by this time.

In the first study, 50% of those who relapsed after abrupt withdrawal did so within 2–10 weeks. Since lithium is completely eliminated from the body in approximately seven days, the high relapse rate over the timeframe described cannot be exclusively a 'drug withdrawal' effect. In the light of this evidence, it would seem prudent always to withdraw lithium treatment gradually, over at least four weeks (if not longer).

Patients may decide that they wish to stop taking lithium, for a variety of perfectly valid reasons (for example, being well for a long time, lack of effect, side-effects). Abrupt discontinuation clearly adds a substantial and clinically important additional risk of early relapse. NH should be advised to recommence lithium immediately, and then either continue with treatment or discontinue gradually after a full discussion of the potential risks and benefits to her and her planned baby.

3. What problems might be anticipated when lithium is taken during pregnancy?
Lithium is known to cross the placenta readily and cases of neonatal cardiac arrhythmia, hypotonia and hypothyroidism have been reported (see review by Schou, 1990). A raised incidence of foetal malformations caused by exposure in the first trimester has also been reported and lithium is widely considered to be a teratogen. This is largely because the Danish register of lithium babies, which was operated on a system of retrospective voluntary reporting, found that 25 of the first 225 births recorded were associated with major congenital malformations. Ebstein's anomaly (a rare congenital downward displacement of the tricuspid valve

into the right ventricle) was found in six of these babies and other cardiac abnormalities in a further 12 (Frankenberg and Lipinski, 1983). However, retrospective voluntary reporting attracts a disproportionate number of adverse outcomes and it is impossible to quantify the risks of lithium without knowing the total number of babies exposed and the number of adverse outcomes that were not reported. A more recent 148-patient prospective study (Jacobson et al, 1992) found that congenital malformation rates with lithium (2.8%) were similar to control rates (2.4%) and suggested that lithium is not an important human teratogen. It should be noted, however, that one case of Ebstein's anomaly was diagnosed at 16 weeks' gestation in the fetus of a patient taking lithium and the pregnancy was terminated. Also, echocardiographs were performed in less than half of the babies born, and so it is possible that minor cardiac defects went undetected.

This study would suggest that lithium is not as teratogenic as is widely believed. The authors suggest that, provided level II ultrasound and fetal echocardiography are performed, women exposed to lithium during pregnancy should not be at undue risk of an adverse outcome. It is also of interest that 21 of the lithium-exposed babies in this study were followed up after birth. They did not differ from a control group in their achievement of major developmental milestones. Nevertheless, the situation is far from clear and the teratogenic potential of lithium remains uncertain. Some caution is obviously required.

Another important consideration is that renal clearance is increased during pregnancy and higher doses of lithium may be required to maintain therapeutic serum levels. Thus, regular close monitoring is essential. Particular care should be taken around the time of delivery, as changes in fluid balance can lead to sudden changes in plasma levels, placing both the mother and the neonate at risk. Some prescribers choose to stop lithium before delivery and restart within 48 hours in order to minimise both the risks above and the risk of relapse in the mother. It is not always possible to plan with such precision.

Some sensible guidelines on the use of lithium in pregnancy are included in an article by Cohen et al (1994).

Key points

- Long-term lithium prophylaxis markedly reduces the excess mortality of people with recurrent affective disorders.
- Although subject to debate, it is unlikely that those who discontinue treatment with lithium will subsequently fail to respond.
- The risk of recurrence of mania may be up to 28 times higher in the first three months after lithium is stopped than it is for those who continue with treatment. This recurrence rate may exceed that of untreated bipolar illness.
- Relapse rates are greater after abrupt withdrawal (1–14 days) than gradual withdrawal (15–30 days).
- Lithium readily crosses the placenta and dose-related side-effects may occur in the neonate.
- Lithium may not be as teratogenic as is commonly believed.
- The risk of fetal cardiac malformations cannot be excluded and all women exposed to lithium in pregnancy should undergo level II ultrasound and fetal echocardiography.

References

Baldessarini RJ, Tondo L, Faedda GL et al (1996) Effects of the rate of discontinuing lithium maintenance treatment in bipolar disorders, *J Clin Psychiatry* **57**: 441–8.

Baldessarini RJ, Tondo L, Floris G et al (1997) Reduced morbidity after gradual discontinuation of lithium treatment for bipolar I and II disorders: a replication study, *Am J Psychiatry* **154**: 551–3.

Bauer M (1994) Refractoriness induced by lithium discontinuation despite adequate serum lithium levels, *Am J Psychiatry* **151**: 1522.

Berghofer A, Kossmann B, Muller-Oerlinghausen B (1996) Course of illness and pattern of recurrence in patients with affective disorders during long-term lithium prophylaxis: a retrospective analysis over 15 years, *Acta Psychiatr Scand* **93**: 349–54.

Cohen LS, Friedman JM, Jefferson JW et al (1994) A re-evaluation of risk of in utero exposure to lithium, *J Am Med Assoc* **271**: 146–50.

Frankenberg FR, Lipinski JF (1983) Congenital malformations, *N Eng J Med* **309**: 311–12.

Gershon S, Soares JC (1997) Current therapeutic profile of lithium, *Arch Gen Psychiatry* **54**: 16–20.

Goodwin G (1995) Lithium revisited. A re-examination of the placebo-controlled trials of lithium prophylaxis in manic-depressive disorder, *Br J Psychiatry* **167:** 573–4.

Jacobson SJ, Jones K, Johnson K et al (1992) Prospective multicentre study of pregnancy outcome after lithium exposure during first trimester, *Lancet* **339:** 530–3.

Johnson RE, McFarland BH (1996) Lithium use and discontinuation in a health maintenance organization, *Am J Psychiatry* **153:** 993–1000.

Maj M, Pirozzi R, Magliano L (1995) Nonresponse to reinstituted lithium prophylaxis in previously responsive bipolar patients: prevalence and predictors, *Am J Psychiatry* **152:** 1810–1.

Muller-Oerlinghausen B, Wolf T, Ahrens B et al (1996) Mortality of patients who dropped out from regular lithium prophylaxis: a collaborative study by the International Group for the Study of Lithium-treated patients (IGSLI). *Acta Psychiatr Scand* **94:** 344–7.

Schou M (1990) Lithium treatment during pregnancy, delivery, and lactation: an update, *J Clin Psychiatry* **51:** 410–13.

Suppes T, Baldessarini RJ, Faedda GL et al (1991) Risk of recurrence following discontinuation of lithium treatment in bipolar disorder, *Arch Gen Psychiatry* **48:** 1082–8.

Tondo L, Baldessarini RJ, Floris G et al (1997) Effectiveness of restarting lithium treatment after its discontinuation in bipolar I and bipolar II disorders, *Am J Psychiatry* **154:** 548–50.

Rapid-cycling bipolar affective disorder

David Taylor

20

SC, a 33-year-old woman with a long history of bipolar affective disorder, including 11 previous hospital admissions, has currently been an inpatient for three months.

SC has not been observed to be euthymic throughout this period. Her mood changes rapidly from hypomania (characterised by sexual disinhibition and grandiosity) to depression and back again. Each period lasts only a few days. When depressed, SC ruminates about suicide and needs almost constant nursing observation. She has made two suicide attempts since being admitted, on one occasion drinking bleach and on another running head-first into a solid wall.

Her current medication is as follows:

Lithium carbonate (as Priadel)	1200 mg at night
Lofepramine	210 mg at night
Carbamazepine	200 mg twice daily

Questions

1. How might treatment be optimised?
2. What other drug alternatives are available?
3. Which 'experimental' therapies might be used in severe, refractory rapid cycling?

Answers

1. How might treatment be optimised?

SC is suffering from rapid-cycling bipolar affective disorder. This is usually defined by the occurrence of four or more episodes of hypomania or depression during a 12-month period (Dunner and Fieve, 1974). Up to 20% of bipolar patients presenting for treatment may have rapid-cycling illness (Coryell et al, 1992), and it is more common in females. Rapid cycling is notoriously difficult to treat effectively.

Both pharmacological and non-pharmacological factors are associated with rapid cycling. Of these, the use of antidepressants, especially tricyclic antidepressants, is perhaps the most important: these drugs have frequently been implicated as precipitants of rapid cycling (Persad et al, 1996). However,

it should be noted that this has been disputed by Coryell et al (1992), who followed up prospectively a cohort of 919 patients with major affective disorders over a five-year period. Forty-five patients developed a rapid-cycling illness during the first year of this study and the authors concluded that the use of tricyclics or MAOIs did not predict rapid cycling (after statistical control for the presence of major depression had been employed). They postulated that it is the episode of major depression that is predictive of the switch into rapid cycling, rather than the treatment that is administered (a so-called epiphenomenon).

Nevertheless, a logical first step in optimising therapy for SC would be the withdrawal of lofepramine. Subsequent depressive episodes should be treated by psychological means, whenever possible.

Lithium, it has been suggested (Dunner and Fieve, 1974), is often ineffective in rapid cycling when used alone. However, there is some evidence to suggest that lithium given with carbamazepine shows synergy, at least in the treatment of mania (Lipinski and Pope, 1982; Kramlinger and Post, 1989). Lithium should therefore be continued and the dose adjusted, if necessary, to give a 12-hour plasma level of 0.6–1.2 mmol/l.

Carbamazepine is commonly used in bipolar disorder and has been shown to be effective in rapid cycling when added to lithium therapy (Joyce, 1988). However, higher doses than 400 mg/day are usually required to produce a therapeutic effect. Indeed, it has been suggested that in bipolar disorder in general, doses of at least 600 mg/day should be used to give plasma levels of above 7 mg/l (Taylor and Duncan, 1997). Thus, a dose increase would be appropriate for SC. Modified-release tablets are better tolerated and should be used. The minimum dose should be that which gives a trough plasma level of 7 mg/l; the maximum dose is best governed by patient tolerability and response, rather than plasma level.

2. What other drug alternatives are available?

In the UK, only lithium and carbamazepine are licensed as mood stabilisers. In the United States, valproate (as divalproex sodium) is also available and widely used. There is some compelling evidence that valproate is effective in rapid cycling when used alone or when added to lithium or carbamazepine, even if these therapies have proved ineffective (e.g. McElroy et al, 1988; Calabrese and Delucchi, 1990; Calabrese et al, 1992). Valproate is therefore often recommended as first- or second-line therapy in rapid cycling, either alone or in combination (Calabrese and Woyshville, 1995; Taylor and Duncan, 1996). Average effective doses are around 1500 mg/day (Taylor and Duncan, 1997). Modified-release tablets seem to be better tolerated than other preparations.

Other drugs available include clozapine, which is effective in treatment-refractory mania (Calabrese et al, 1996) and appears to have some activity in rapid cycling (Suppes et al, 1994). Clozapine is licensed in the UK only for treatment-refractory schizophrenia, although the manufacturers are sympathetic to requests for 'out of licence' use and consider each case individually.

Thyroxine also seems effective in rapid cycling (Taylor and Duncan, 1996), although it should be noted that this is as an add-on to existing therapy. In some cases, efficacy has been shown when thyroxine has been used as an adjunct to antidepressants, fuelling the debate mentioned above (Bauer and Whybrow, 1990). Clonazepam may be effective in the maintenance treatment of bipolar disorder (Sachs et al, 1990). However, it should be noted that none of these treatments has been comprehensively evaluated and definitively shown to be effective. Further studies are needed and caution is advised when these medications are used.

3. Which 'experimental' therapies might be used in severe, refractory rapid cycling?

Rapid cycling is so often unresponsive to standard treatments that many other putative, experimental therapies have been investigated. They include nimodipine, lamotrigine and gabapentin, None is officially licensed for use in bipolar disorder and none has been robustly evaluated in rapid cycling. Nevertheless, these experimental drugs are frequently used as a last resort in refractory cases. Despite the inherent unresponsiveness of these patients, a worthwhile response is sometimes observed.

Nimodipine is a centrally acting calcium antagonist usually used in the treatment of subarachnoid haemorrhage. A small double-blind trial first suggested activity (Pazzaglia et al, 1993) and this finding has subsequently been supported by case reports (Goodnick, 1995). Doses of 30–60 mg tds are initially used and may be effective. Up to 360 mg/day has been used. Adverse effects are infrequent and trivial.

Lamotrigine is a relatively new anticonvulsant which has for some time been considered potentially useful in mood disorders. Calabrese et al (1996) were the first to report a case of response to the drug in rapid cycling. Antidepressant effects were particularly evident. Other case series have since been reported. Kusumakar and Yatham (1997) reported successful treatment in four of seven rapid-cycling patients and Sporn and Sachs (1997) described good outcome in eight of 16 patients with refractory bipolar disorder (four of the eight were rapid cyclers). Slow introduction of lamotrigine is essential to avoid rash. Doses in responders average around 150 mg/day.

Gabapentin, another recently introduced anticonvulsant, may also be effective. At least two case series have been published (Bennett et al, 1997; Schaffer and Schaffer, 1997), broadly indicating good activity in refractory mood disorders. Neither report provided much information relating specifically to rapid cycling. Obviously, further studies are required.

Case reports and open studies of experimental treatments should be interpreted with due consideration of the prognosis of rapid-cycling illness. The study by Coryell et al (1992) found that, while patients with rapid-cycling illness had a significant lower likelihood of recovery in the second year of follow-up, the prognosis improved significantly after this time, with only one of 45 patients exhibiting a rapid-cycling illness for the entire five-year follow-up period. The remission rate was high in years 3 to 5, and so case reports featuring patients apparently 'responding' at this stage in their illness should be treated with particular caution.

Key points

- Up to 20% of bipolar patients presenting for treatment have had four or more episodes of hypomania or depression during the previous 12 months (rapid cycling).
- Antidepressants may precipitate rapid cycling.
- Lithium is often ineffective when used alone, but may offer benefit in combination with carbamazepine.
- Sodium valproate may be effective, either alone or in combination with lithium or carbamazepine.
- Unlicensed options worth considering in patients with refractory illness include thyroxine, clozapine, nimodipine, lamotrigine and gabapentin.
- Patients with rapid-cycling illness have a poor prognosis in the short term, but it is likely that only a very small proportion continue to cycle rapidly for more than a few years.

References

Bauer M, Whybrow PC (1990) Rapid cycling bipolar affective disorder II. Treatment of refractory rapid cycling with high dose levothyroxine. A preliminary study, *Arch Gen Psych* **47**: 435–40.

Bennett J, Goldman WT, Suppes T (1997) Gabapentin for treatment of bipolar and schizoaffective disorders, *J Clin Psychopharmacol* **17**: 141–2.

Calabrese JR, Delucchi GA (1990) Spectrum of efficacy of valproate in 55 patients with rapid-cycling bipolar disorder, *Am J Psychiatry* **147:** 431–4.

Calabrese JR, Fatemi SH, Woyshville MJ (1996) Antidepressant effects of lamotrigine in rapid cycling bipolar disorder, *Am J Psychiatry* **153:** 1236.

Calabrese JR, Kimmel SE, Woyshville MJ et al (1996) Clozapine for treatment-refractory mania, *Am J Psychiatry* **153:** 759–64.

Calabrese JR, Markovitz PJ, Kimmel SE et al (1992) Spectrum of efficacy of valproate in 78 Rapid-cycling bipolar patients, *J Clin Psychopharmacol* **12:** 53S–56S.

Calabrese JR, Woyshville MJ (1995) A medication algorithm for treatment of bipolar rapid cycling? *J Clin Psychiatry* **56:** 11–18.

Coryell W, Endicott J, Keller M (1992) Rapidly cycling affective disorder: demographics, diagnosis, family history, and course, *Arch Gen Psychiatry* **49:** 126–31.

Dunner DL, Fieve RR (1974) Clinical factors in lithium carbonate prophylaxis failure, *Arch Gen Psychiatry* **30:** 229–33.

Goodnick PJ (1995) Nimodipine treatment of rapid cycling bipolar disorder, *J Clin Psych* **56:** 330.

Joyce PR (1988) Carbamazepine in rapid cycling bipolar affective disorder, *Int Clin Psychopharmacol* **3:** 123–9.

Kramlinger KG, Post RM (1989) Adding lithium carbonate to carbamazepine: antimanic efficacy in treatment-resistant mania, *Acta Psychiatr Scand* **79:** 378–85.

Kusumakar V, Yatham LN (1997) Lamotrigine treatment of rapid cycling bipolar disorder, *Am J Psychiatry* **154:** 1171–2.

Lipinski JF, Pope HG Jr (1982) Possible synergistic action between carbamazepine and lithium carbonate in the treatment of three acutely manic patients, *Am J Psychiatry* **139:** 948–9.

McElroy SL, Keck PE Jr, Pope HG et al (1988) Valproate in the treatment of rapid-cycling bipolar disorder, *J Clin Psychopharmacol* **8:** 275–9.

Pazzaglia PJ, Post RM, Ketter TA (1993) Preliminary controlled trial of nimodipine in ultra-rapid cycling affective dysregulation, *Psychiatry Res* **49:** 257–72.

Persad E, Oluboka OJ, Sharma V et al (1996) The phenomenon of rapid cycling in bipolar mood disorders: a review, *Can J Psychiatry* **41:** 23–7.

Sachs GS, Rosenbaum JR, Jones L (1990) Adjunctive clonazepam for maintenance treatment of bipolar affective disorder, *J Clin Psychopharmacol* **10:** 42–7.

Schaffer CB, Schaffer LC (1997) Gabapentin in the treatment of bipolar disorder, *Am J Psychiatry* **154:** 291–2.

Sporn J, Sachs G (1997) The anticonvulsant lamotrigine in treatment-resistant manic-depressive illness, *J Clin Psychopharmacol* **17:** 185–9.

Suppes T, Phillips KA, Judd CR (1994) Clozapine treatment of nonpsychotic rapid cycling bipolar disorder: a report of three cases, *Biol Psychiatry* **36:** 338–40.

Taylor D, Duncan D (1996) Treatment options for rapid-cycling bipolar affective disorder, *Psychiatr Bull* **20:** 601–3.

Taylor D, Duncan D (1997) Doses of carbamazepine and valproate in bipolar affective disorder, *Psychiatr Bull* **21:** 221–3.

Bipolar disorder: unlicensed treatments

Peter Pratt

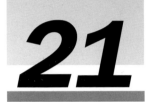

AS, a 45-year-old unemployed baker, had been admitted to an acute psychiatric ward some three months previously following a deterioration in his relationship with his partner of ten years.

During this admission, ward staff noted frequent episodes of sexual disinhibition. At other times he appeared weepy and apologetic. Occupational therapy staff reported his very short attention span and inability to concentrate. His sleep pattern varied considerably but he frequently reported little need for sleep.

AS first presented to the psychiatric services six years ago following referral by his GP. He presented with poor appetite and sleep disturbance, was very weepy, felt unable to cope and could not face going to work. He felt his workmates were trying to get him sacked by putting insects or glass in the bread he baked. These symptoms were well controlled by fluoxetine

20 mg/day and trifluoperazine 10 mg/day. A year later, AS was admitted to an acute psychiatric ward: his partner had become unhappy at his increasingly frequent and bizarre sexual demands. At the time he also believed she had become a prostitute and would be able to access all the other prostitutes in the city. A diagnosis of mania was made and AS was successfully treated with lithium carbonate.

Over the next four years AS had five further psychiatric admissions, one for a depressive episode and four due to mania. Both AS and his partner confirmed that he regularly took lithium and blood levels confirmed a reasonably steady 12-hour level of around 0.6–0.8 mmol/l. Twelve months before his current admission lithium was discontinued and carbamazepine started in an attempt to prevent further episodes.

Extensive medical and neurobiological investigations have found no abnormalities. AS does not normally drink alcohol and has not misused drugs for at least 20 years. In the past he had taken various illicit substances, particularly magic mushrooms and anabolic steroids.

AS's current diagnosis is bipolar affective disorder, manic episode. He is treated with haloperidol 9 mg daily (occasionally up to 15 mg), procyclidine 5 mg twice daily, temazepam up to 20 mg at night and carbamazepine 1,600 mg/day (as 600 mg, 400 mg and 600 mg). There are no grounds to suspect non-compliance with medication. Serum carbamazepine levels are between 10 and 12 mg/l. In retrospect, AS feels that lithium did not help at all; it just reduced his sex drive.

In view of his apparent non-response to lithium or carbamazepine, AS is asked to consider taking sodium valproate – an unlicensed treatment.

Questions

1. What is meant by an unlicensed treatment?
2. What are the implications for prescribers of using unlicensed treatment and in what framework should it be done?
3. What are the pharmacological treatment options and what would be the treatment of choice in AS?

Answers

1. What is meant by an unlicensed treatment?

In the UK, the Medicines Control Agency (MCA) is the main body that must be satisfied that a medicine is both safe and effective for its intended use. In order to reach this conclusion, the MCA will require a manufacturer to submit supporting data demonstrating the effects of the medicine. The MCA considers animal data (from preclinical studies), healthy volunteer data (usually phase I clinical studies) and patient data (usually phase II and III studies). Preclinical studies may employ animal models of human disease states and are also concerned with acute and chronic toxicity. Early clinical studies are concerned with determining the drug's clinical pharmacokinetics. Dose-finding studies follow, and then randomised, placebo-controlled, double-blind trials

in patients. Many of the patients treated routinely in clinical practice are excluded from clinical trials, e.g. the elderly, those who have significant physical pathology, or those who cannot give informed consent. If a manufacturer wants to extend the use of a licensed drug, similar supporting evidence for the intended new use must be provided to the MCA. If, then, the MCA is satisfied that a new medicine or a new use of an existing medicine is safe, effective and brings about overall benefit, then the licensing authority (Ministry of Health) will grant a *Product Licence*. Health economic (cost effectiveness) data are not currently required by the MCA.

Following the setting up of the European Medicines Evaluation Agency (EMEA) in 1995, the process of granting Product Licences has been co-ordinated across the European Union.

If a licence is granted in one country, it is expected that this would be recognised in other member states.

Any drug that has not been granted a product licence is termed an unlicensed product. Also, the use of licensed medicines in conditions or · dose schedules not included in their licence is officially unlicensed use (sometimes called 'off label').

Sodium valproate is licensed for the treatment of epilepsy, but if used for the management of bipolar disorder it would be considered an unlicensed treatment. (Even though valproate as Divalproex does have a licence for use in mania associated with bipolar disorder in the USA.)

2. What are the implications for prescribers of using unlicensed treatments and in what framework should it be done?

Few people outside the licensing process will know the full details of a product licence. From a practical point of view, the information required to prescribe within a licence will be contained within the medicine's summary of product characteristic (SPC). Previously this was referred to as a data sheet. The majority of SPCs are contained in the data sheet

compendium which is published annually by the ABPI. (Manufacturers who are not members of ABPI will not have their SPC included in this text.)

If a drug is prescribed, there is an expectation that this is done knowingly, that is, with an appreciation of information contained in the SPC. If no reference is made to the SPC it may be alleged that the prescriber was negligent (Anon, 1992).

However, doctors may still reasonably prescribe unlicensed medicines or use medicines outside their product licence. Warnings and special precautions may be overridden. Advice may also be given to other prescribers to use a product in an unlicensed way. Responsibility for adverse effects may then lie entirely with the prescriber, however.

Drugs that have no product licence for any indication must be obtained on a 'named-patient' basis, before they can be supplied to a patient. Such drugs are not routinely stocked in any pharmacy. Pharmaceutical manufacturers may supply a product for a 'named patient', but it is important to emphasise that it is the prescriber who bears all responsibility for its use.

Licensing, or extending a licence, is an expensive process. It may be uneconomic for a manufacturer to apply for a licence extension to cover a small-scale, specialist use of a product. This is why many drugs continue to have a narrow range of official indications, despite use in other conditions.

If called to justify the unlicensed use of a drug, a prescriber may find it helpful to point to standard texts such as the British National Formulary (BNF) if they support the use in practice. Widely held clinical opinion as voiced in consensus statements, or Royal College guidelines, are another source of support.

As a general principle an unlicensed treatment should not be used in place of an effective and well-tolerated licensed treatment (the licensing process is thus in effect supporting the use of evidence-based pharmaco-therapy). In psychiatric practice there are often a significant number of patients who show a limited or partial response to existing treatments. Considering this, together with some of the disabling side-effects of many psychiatric drugs, the use of unlicensed treatments is understandable and often justifiable.

The prescriber should always clearly document the reasons for prescribing in the clinical notes. He or she may be wise to seek a second opinion.

Wherever possible the prescriber and/or the pharmacist should explain to the patient that they are receiving an unlicensed treatment and the impli-cations that this may have. With the increased availability of standard infor-mation in packs of medicines a patient may be particularly confused if the literature in their medicine makes no reference to their condition.

3. What are the pharmacological treatment options and what would be the treatment of choice in AS?

AS has been treated with 9–15 mg haloperidol/day for the duration of his current admission. Depending on the manufacturer, the licensed daily dose for haloperidol is up to 100 mg (120 mg rarely in resistant schizophre-nia) although there appears little ratio-nale for increasing the dose above 10 mg (Rifkin et al, 1994). The summary product characteristic (SPC) from the two manufacturers of haloperidol and the BNF are consistent, in that they both suggest daily doses of around 10 mg to 15 mg (BNF, 1997; Walker, 1996). Increasing the dose above 120 mg/day would normally be considered an unlicensed use. In anything other than exceptional cases, the use of antipsychotics in such an unlicensed way would not be supported by informed clinical opinion (Thompson, 1994).

Carbamazepine is licensed for use in epilepsy in daily doses of up to 2000 mg/day. In the prophylaxis of bipolar disorder 1600 mg is the maximum licensed daily dose. Little evidence exists to support the use of carbamazepine in doses above this. Simhandl and colleagues (1993) found no difference in prophylactic efficacy in bipolar patients with low or high serum levels of carbamazepine. There appears no justification for exceeding the licensed dose in this case.

Sodium valproate is not licensed for use in bipolar disorder in the UK. As divalproex it is approved for use in the treatment of mania associated with bipolar disorder in the USA. Divalproex is an equimolar combination of sodium valproate and valproic acid. (For a comprehensive review of valproic acid see Balfour and Bryson (1994).)

The evidence supporting the use of valproate as prophylaxis in bipolar affective disorder and schizoaffective disorder originates mostly from open studies that do not include a placebo arm. In both the treatment of mania and the prevention of manic relapse, the evidence, although limited, appears more robust (Silverstone and Romans, 1996; Ahmed and Morriss, 1997). In the treatment of mania the response rate appears to be similar to lithium, at around 50% (Bowden et al, 1994; Bowden, 1996). Data from a multicentre, double-blind study of 179 hospitalised manic patients suggests that those with depressive symptoms at baseline were less likely to respond to lithium than to divalproex (Swann et al, 1997). Although the overall response rate appeared similar, the authors suggest that lithium and divalproex may be effective in clinically and biologically distinct groups. These conclusions should be confirmed by further studies before they are considered definitive.

In view of AS's predominant manic symptoms and failure to respond to established licensed treatment, a good case can be made to support treatment with sodium valproate. There is no consensus on dosage. Ahmed and Morriss (1997) suggest treatment should be started at 250 mg two or three times daily and then increased by 250–500 mg every three days to a maximum dose of 60 mg/kg per day. The dose should be adjusted according to side-effects and response. Patients suffering gastrointestinal intolerance from conventional tablets may be switched to the slow-release form, which is usually better tolerated.

There is no linear relationship between plasma level and response (Bowden, 1996). Taylor and Duncan's review (1997) concurs with others in advising that plasma levels above 50 mg/l are required for a therapeutic response. Side-effects seem more common with levels above 100 mg/l.

If AS responds to valproate, long-term treatment would be justified. If valproate is ineffective, other unlicensed treatments may be considered for AS.

Case reports and open studies provide limited evidence for the benefit of lamotrigine and gabapentin both as individual agents and in combination with lithium (Freeman and Stoll, 1998).

Benzodiazepines may have a role over and above any sedating or tranquillising effect. Lorazepam is frequently used in mania as an adjunct to other treatments where its primary role is in reducing the need for additional doses of antipsychotic. Some published evidence also supports the use of clonazepam, although the small number of cases and use of drug combinations make it difficult to conclude that clonazepam has a specific antimanic effect. Chouinard and colleagues (1983) found clonazepam to be as effective overall as lithium, but superior in controlling hyperactivity.

There is a reasonable theoretical base for using calcium channel blocking agents in bipolar disorder. Elevated levels of calcium ions have been found in both platelets and lymphocytes of manic and depressed bipolar patients. Of the calcium channel blockers, verapamil is the best supported by double-blind, placebo-controlled studies as well as open studies and case reports. The available evidence suggests that verapamil in doses around 240 mg to 480 mg is effective in the treatment of mania. Unlike valproate and carbamazepine, verapamil may not be as effective in lithium-resistant cases. Overall there are insufficient data to conclude that verapamil is as effective as lithium. Walton and colleagues (1996) in their single-blind study of 40 manic patients found lithium to be a superior treatment.

The evidence supporting two other calcium channel blockers, nifedipine and nimodipine, is limited. Given that these drugs may act at different binding sites in the brain, individual calcium antagonists may prove to have benefits over and above their 'class effects'. The prophylactic effect of calcium antagonists is yet to be determined. Adverse effects such as hypotension and constipation are often dose-limiting, especially with verapamil.

Drug combinations may also be used. In an attempt to quantify the risks and benefits of drug combination in the treatment of bipolar disorder. Freeman and Stoll (1998) reviewed the published evidence and concluded that the safest and most effective mood stabiliser combinations were anticonvulsants, particularly sodium valproate, with lithium.

Many other unlicensed treatments have been tried in bipolar disorder (Lerer, 1985), but their use should be considered limited. Effective non-pharmacological strategies, such as ECT (electroconvulsive therapy) should not be discounted in favour of these obscure treatments. Several of the atypical antipsychotics have also been used, mainly in combination with lithium. The absence of extrapyramidal problems would justify further work in identifying the role of these agents in bipolar disorder.

Key points

- Satisfactory evidence of both safety and efficacy is required before the MCA will issue a product licence.
- The licensing process is the 'evidence' in evidence-based pharmacotherapy.
- When a drug is prescribed for an unlicensed use, the prescriber usually bears full responsibility for any adverse consequence.
- Patients should be informed when they are prescribed a drug for an unlicensed indication.
- Support for the use of a drug for an unlicensed indication may be found in the BNF, or may take the form of widely held clinical opinion voiced in consensus statements.
- Sodium valproate is not licensed in the UK for the treatment of bipolar disorder.

References

Ahmed M, Morriss R (1997) Assessment and management of rapid cycling bipolar affective disorder, *Adv Psychiatr Treat* **3:** 367–73.

Anon (1992) Prescribing unlicenced drugs or using drugs for unlicenced indications, *Drug Thera Bull* **30:** 97–100.

Balfour JA, Bryson HM (1994) Valproic acid: a review of its pharmacology and therapeutic potential in indications other than epilepsy, *CNS Drugs* **2:** 144–73.

Bowden CL (1996) Dosing strategies and time course of response to antimanic drugs, *J Clin Psychiatry* **57:** (Suppl. 13), 4–9.

Bowden CL, Brugger AM, Swann AC et al (1994) Efficacy of divalproex sodium vs lithium and placebo in the treatment of mania, *J Am Med Assoc* **271:** 918–24.

British National Formulary, 34 (1997) London, UK: British Medical Association and Royal Pharmaceutical Society of Great Britain.

Chouinard G, Young SN, Annable L (1983) Antimanic effects of clonazepam, *Biol Psychiatry* **18:** 451–66.

Freeman MP, Stoll AL (1998) Mood stabilizer combinations: a review of safety and efficacy, *Am J Psychiatry* **155:** 12–21.

Lerer B (1985) Alternative therapies for bipolar disorder, *J Clin Psychiatry* **46:** 309–16.

Rifkin A, Doddi S, Karajgi B et al (1994) Dosage of haloperidol for mania, *Br J Psychiatry* **165:** 113–16.

Silverstone T, Romans S (1996) Long-term treatment of bipolar disorder, *Drugs* **51:** 367–82.

Simhandl C, Denk E, Thau K (1993) The comparative efficacy of carbamazepine at low and high serum levels and lithium carbonate in the prophylaxis of affective disorders, *J Affect Disord* **28:** 221–31.

Swann AC, Bowden CL, Morris D et al (1997) Depression during mania. Treatment response to lithium or divalproex, *Arch Gen Psych* **54**(1) 37–42.

Taylor D, Duncan D (1997) Doses of carbamazepine and valproate in bipolar affective disorder, *Psych Bull* **21:** 221–23.

Thompson C (1994) The use of high dose antipsychotic medication, *Br J Psychiatry* **164:** 448–58.

Walker G (1996) *ABPI Compendium of Data Sheets and Summaries of Product Characteristics.* (London: Datapharm Publications).

Walton SA, Berk M, Brook S (1996) Superiority of lithium over verapamil in mania: a randomised controlled, single blind trial, *J Clin Psychiatry* **57:** 543–5.

Self-injurious behaviour and learning disabilities

Dave Branford

22

KH, is a 30-year-old severely learning-disabled woman. She is the youngest of three children. Both her brother and sister are of normal intelligence and free from any mental illness. The cause of KH's learning disability is unknown. From an early age KH showed autistic behaviours and was diagnosed as suffering from childhood autism. She suffered a first seizure at the age of 11 and a second, which may have been secondary to high lithium levels, at the age of 15 years.

The following are a series of situations that have occurred with KH over the years.

At the age of 14 KH was admitted permanently to hospital. Her behaviour had dramatically deteriorated following a series of changes at home and attempts at short-term breaks in hospital. She was biting herself and others, ripping her clothes and bedding and banging her head repeatedly. She was receiving carbamazepine 200 mg twice daily at this time.

Since admission to hospital KH has remained difficult to control. Her self-injurious behaviours continue to be extreme in severity. Repeated attempts at short-term breaks failed and her parents did not feel they could cope with her any more. Treatment with an increased dose of carbamazepine did not bring any benefit, and large doses of chlorpromazine resulted only in short-term drowsiness. Ten years on, KH still presents with a wide variety of self-injurious and destructive behaviours. These include: biting herself mostly on her shoulders and knee, slapping herself, pulling her own hair and banging her head. Occasionally she will bite others, attempt to pull their fingers back, obsessionally put her head down the toilet or attempt to flush her clothes down the toilet, scream, smash windows using her hand or head and deliberately urinate in bed. Throughout this period she has remained on carbamazepine 300 mg bd, lithium carbonate 500 mg BD and

fluctuating doses of chlorpromazine. At one point, when these behaviours were at their most severe, chlorpromazine was prescribed at a dose of 1 g daily.

Physical examination revealed significant scarring to many areas of the body. Full blood count, thyroid function and urea and electrolyte tests were unremarkable, although both a tremor and an orofacial dyskinesia were evident. Her serum lithium level was 0.9 mmol/l.

The EEG report states:
    The record contains a fair
    amount of alpha activity at
    8–9 Hz, 20–50 µV reactive and
    symmetrical. A fair amount of
    theta activity is present at
    20–24 Hz, up to 35 µV inter-
    mixed and superimposed. No
    focal activity is found.
    Conclusion: The background is
    mildly abnormal. There are no
    focal/paroxysmal features seen.

Questions

1. What possible psychological, social and biological theories could explain the continued self-injury?
2. Give the arguments for and against the continuation of the carbamazepine.
3. Give the arguments for and against the continuation of the lithium carbonate.
4. Give the arguments for and against the continued prescribing of an antipsychotic drug.
5. What alternative drug therapies may be of benefit?

Answers

1. What possible psychological, social and biological theories could explain the continued self-injury?

Self-injurious behaviour (SIB) is a devastating and chronic problem which, although not exclusively confined to people with learning disabilities, presents a particular problem with this population (Reid and Ballinger, 1995). There is no clear understanding of the aetiology of SIB. Learning theories postulate that the behaviour may be reinforced by rewards such as attention or avoidance, and started by response to an event such as pain, menstruation, level of stimulation or mental illness.

Animal models suggest that SIB may have a biological cause. These include dopamine dysfunction particularly associated with D_1 receptors (Breese et al, 1995; Schroeder et al, 1995) and opiate system dysfunction where SIB results in elevated levels of beta-endorphin. It has been suggested that the latter may be an analogous to an addiction (Sandman and Hetrick, 1995).

2. Give the arguments for and against the continuation of the carbamazepine.

The following questions are relevant to the continuation of carbamazepine, lithium or antipsychotic drugs:

- Is the medicine indicated?
- Is there any evidence that it has been of value?
- Is the patient suffering from any adverse effects?
- Are withdrawal problems likely?

Is carbamazepine indicated? There are two issues to consider: firstly, is carbamazepine indicated for SIB and, secondly, is the patient suffering from active epilepsy? Much of the scarce evidence to support the use of carbamazepine for SIB is equivocal. For example, Barrett et al (1988) reported the use of carbamazepine in an 11-year-old girl with mild learning disabilities and epilepsy and found that, although self-injury, growling noises and facial grimacing were reduced, other unacceptable maladaptive behaviours were not. The second issue of whether antiepileptic drug treatment remains indicated for a person with severe learning disabilities when there has been no record of seizures for over ten years remains difficult. The EEG result supports the decision to withdraw the carbamazepine. Also there is not really any evidence that the carbamazepine has been of value.

Carbamazepine is associated with many side-effects including nausea, ataxia and drowsiness.

Although there is no withdrawal syndrome associated with carbamazepine, withdrawal may present a problem, particularly as KH has received the drug for many years. A slow programme of gradual withdrawal over a three to six-month period should be recommended.

3. Give the arguments for and against the continuation of the lithium carbonate.
Is lithium indicated? The literature to support the use of lithium to treat aggression, self-mutilation and affective disorders in the context of learning disabilities was reviewed by Johnson (1988), who found the literature to be scant. In two large clinical trials (Tyrer et al, 1984; Craft et al, 1987) no clear opinion on the value of lithium treatment for SIB was developed. Most of the papers to support the efficacy of lithium were open trials involving small numbers of patients. For example, Micev and Lynch (1974) had earlier found that lithium had produced complete elimination of SIB in six of eight self-mutilating patients. The literature to support the use of lithium for affective disorders is large but there is no indication in this case that the patient is suffering from an affective disorder.

There is no evidence that lithium has been of any value in this patient. The treatment has continued for almost 10 years, during which time the SIB has remained similar in frequency and severity. KH has received an adequate dose and there is some evidence that she is suffering from side-effects, notably tremor.

Although there are not usually any withdrawal effects associated with the use of lithium in SIB, it would be advisable to reduce the dose slowly over a three-month period.

4. Give the arguments for and against the continued prescribing of an antipsychotic drug.
Antipsychotic drugs have historically been the drugs most widely prescribed for SIB although the evidence to support their efficacy is largely anecdotal. The suggestion that SIB can be more effectively treated by antipsychotic drugs which have a high affinity for the dopamine D1 receptor rather than dopamine D2 was first proposed by Breese et al (1990) and subsequently tested by Schroeder et al (1995) using fluphenazine. Support for this hypothesis had also come from Hammock et al (1995), who studied the use of clozapine, an antipsychotic drug with a high affinity for D1 receptors, for SIB.

There has been only a limited effect of the antipsychotic drug chlorpromazine in this patient, even at high doses. The

change to a new antipsychotic drug such as olanzapine or quetiapine may be considered, although evidence for their efficacy in this condition is lacking. Chlorpromazine is associated with tardive dyskinesia and tremor. KH is currently suffering from both, although an association is not certain.

There are withdrawal effects associated with antipsychotic drugs. Short-term withdrawal effects such as nausea and vomiting have been associated with antipsychotic drugs that have anticholinergic properties, such as thioridazine and chlorpromazine (Lacoursiere et al, 1976). Other long-term withdrawal effects such as worsening of tardive dyskinesia may also influence both the speed of withdrawal and the likelihood of success. Reduction of dose is more likely to be achievable than total withdrawal (Branford, 1996a; Branford, 1996b).

5. What alternative drug therapies may be of benefit?
A number of alternative drug strategies have been proposed for the treatment of SIB. Those with the best evidence in the literature include the opiate antagonist naltrexone, and the selective serotonin re-uptake inhibitors (SSRIs)

fluoxetine and paroxetine. Others such as propranolol, buspirone, sodium valproate and clonidine are supported by case reports only.

The relatively large body of data on naltrexone contains contradictory reports of both success and failure to treat SIB. A series of controlled studies showed significant naltrexone-related reductions in SIB (Barrett et al, 1989; Bernstein et al, 1987; Herman et al, 1987; Sandman et al, 1990) which were dose related. Other studies have failed to find any such naltrexone-related effects (Szymansky et al, 1987; Zingarelli et al, 1992). A recent study by Bodfish et al (1997) found that reduction of SIB was sustained in only two of nine subjects treated.

Much of the support for SSRIs comes from studies of autism. SIB commonly presents in autism and the obsessive nature of the self-injury has led researchers to suggest that drug treatments used to treat obsessive compulsive disorder may be useful. The antidepressants used are predominantly those that affect serotonin re-uptake and include clomipramine and the SSRI fluoxetine. Most reports involve either individual cases or small numbers (Primeau and Fontaine, 1987;

McDougal et al, 1992; Markowitz, 1990; Lewis et al, 1995). Two large studies include those by Garber et al (1992) which involved 11 people and Cook et al (1992) which involved 23 people with autistic disorder and 16 people with learning disabilities.

Garber et al (1992) found clomipramine to be effective in controlling a range of perseverative behaviours such as head-banging, head-slapping, hand-flapping and rocking in 10 out of 11 children, while McDougal et al (1992) achieved similar success with four out of five young adults with autistic disorder. Cook et al (1992) found fluoxetine at daily doses ranging from 20 mg to 80 mg led to significant improvement in 10 out of 16 individuals with learning disabilities and 15 of 23 individuals with autistic disorder. The absence of total response indicates that no drug treatment is a 'magic bullet' in SIB.

Clinical audit

Although no drug treatment is a 'magic bullet' in SIB, at least 10% of adults with learning disabilities living in the community are prescribed psychotropic drugs (Clarke et al, 1990). Clinical

standards concerning the documentation of the rationale for treatment,
consent and the requirement for regular
psychiatrist review of efficacy and side-
effects can be set. Clinical audit can
then be used to improve prescribing
practice (Miller et al, 1997) in this
vulnerable group of patients who are
unable to articulate their own views.

Key points

- SIB, although not exclusive to
  people with learning disabilities, is
  particularly problematic in this
  population.
- There is no clear understanding of
  the aetiology of SIB.
- Clear documentation of baseline SIB
  is required, along with failure of
  psychological interventions, before
  initiating drug treatment. Attempts
  to monitor the efficacy and side-
  effects of medication should be
  made.
- The objective evidence to support
  the use of carbamazepine, lithium
  and naltrexone in SIB is poor.
- Antipsychotics, particularly those
  with affinity for D_1 receptors, may
  be useful, but side-effects may be
  problematic.
- There is some evidence to support
  the efficacy of SSRIs in SIB.

References

Barrett RP, Feinstein C, Hole WT (1989)
Effects of naloxone and naltrexone on self-
injury: a double blind placebo controlled
analysis, Am J Ment Retard **93**: 644–65.

Barrett RP, Payton JB, Burkhart JE (1988)
Treatment of self-injury and disruptive behaviour with carbamazepine (Tegretol) and
behaviour therapy, J Multihandicapped
Person **1**: 79–91.

Bernstein GA, Hughes JR, Mitchell JE et al
(1987) Effects of narcotic antagonists on
self-injurious behaviour: a single case study,
J Am Acad Child Adolesc Psychiatry **26**:
886–9.

Bodfish JW, McCuller WR, Madison JM et al
(1997) Placebo, double blind evaluation of
long-term naltrexone treatment effects for
adults with mental retardation and self-
injury, J Dev Phys Disabil **9**: 135–53.

Branford D (1996a) A review of antipsychotic drugs prescribed for people with
learning disabilities who live in
Leicestershire, J Intellect Disabil Res **40**:
358–68.

Branford, D (1996b) Factors associated with
the successful or unsuccessful withdrawal of
antipsychotic drug therapy prescribed for
people with learning disabilities, J Intellect
Disabil Res **40**: 322–9.

Breese GR, Criswell HE, Mueller RA (1990) Evidence that lack of brain dopamine during development can increase the susceptibility for aggression and self-injurious behaviour by influencing D1-dopamine receptor function, *Prog Neuropsychopharmacol Biol Psychiatry* **14:** S65–S80.

Breese GR, Criswell HE, Duncan GE et al (1995) Model for reduced brain dopamine in Lesch–Nyhan syndrome and the mentally retarded, *Ment Retard Dev Disabil Res Rev* **1:** 111–19.

Clarke DJ, Kelley S, Thinn K et al (1990) Disabilities and the prescription of drugs for behaviour and for epilepsy in three residential settings, *J Ment Defic Res* **34:** 385–95.

Cook EN, Rowlett R, Jaselskis C et al (1992) Fluoxetine treatment of children and adults with autistic disorder and mental retardation, *J Am Acad Child Adolesc Psychiatry* **31:** 739–45.

Craft M, Ismail IA, Regan A et al (1987) Lithium in the treatment of aggression in mentally handicapped patients: a double blind trial, *Br J Psychiatry* **150:** 685–9.

Garber HJ, McGonigle JJ, Smolka GT et al (1992) Clomipramine treatment of stereotypic behaviours and self-injury in patients with developmental disabilities, *J Am Acad Child Adolesc Psychiatry* **31:** 1157–60.

Hammock RG, Schroeder SR, Levine WR (1995) The effect of clozapine on self-injurious behaviour, *J Autism Dev Disord* **25:** 611–26.

Herman BH, Hammock MK, Smith A et al (1987) Naltrexone decreases self-injurious behaviour, *Ann Neurol* **22:** 550–2.

Johnson FN (1988) Lithium treatment of aggression, self-mutilation and affective disorders in the context of mental handicap, *Reviews Contemporary Pharmacotherapy.* (Carnforth, Lancashire: Marius Press).

Lacoursiere RB, Spohn HE, Thompson K (1976) Medical effects of abrupt neuroleptic withdrawal, *Comprehens Psychiatry* **17:** 285–94.

Lewis MH, Bodfish JW, Powell SB et al (1995) Clomipramine treatment for stereotype and related repetitive movement disorders associated with mental retardation, *Am J Ment Retard* **100:** 299–312.

McDougle CJ, Price LH, Volkman FR et al (1992) Clomipramine in autism: preliminary evidence of efficacy, *J Am Acad Child Adolesc Psychiatry* **31:** 746–50.

Markowitz PI (1990) Fluoxetine treatment of self-injurious behaviour in mentally retarded patients, *J Clin Psychopharmacol* **10:** 299–300.

Micev V, Lynch DM (1974) Effects of lithium on disturbed severely mentally retarded patients, *Br J Psychiatry* **125:** 111.

Miller HE, Simpson N, Foster SE (1997) Psychotropic medication in learning disabilities: audit as an alternative to legislation, *Psychiatr Bull* **21:** 286–9.

Primeau F, Fontaine R (1987) Obsessive disorder with self-mutilation. A subgroup response to pharmacotherapy, *Can J Psychiatry* **32:** 699–701.

Reid AH, Ballinger BR (1995) Behaviour symptoms among severely and profoundly mentally retarded patients. A 16–18 year follow-up study, *Br J Psychiatry* **167:** 452–5.

Sandman CA, Barron JL, Colman H (1990) An orally administered opiate blocker, naltrexone, attenuates self-injurious behaviour, *Am J Ment Retard* **95:** 93–102.

Sandman CA, Hetrick WP (1995) Opiate mechanisms in self-injury, *Ment Retard Dev Disabil Res Rev* **1:** 130–6.

Schroeder SR, Hammock RG, Mulick JA et al (1995) Clinical trials of D_1 and D_2 dopamine modulating drugs and self-injury in mental retardation and developmental disability, *Ment Retard Dev Disabil Res Rev* **1:** 120–9.

Szymanski L, Kekesdy J, Sulkes S et al (1987) Naltrexone in treatment of self-injurious behaviour: a clinical study, *Res Dev Disabil* **8:** 179–90.

Tyrer SP, Walsh A, Edwards DE et al (1984) Factors associated with a good response to lithium in aggressive mentally handicapped subjects, *Prog Neuro-Psychopharmacol* **8:** 755–65.

Zingarelli G, Allman G, Hom A et al (1992) Clinical effects of naltrexone on autistic behaviour, *Am J Ment Retard* **97:** 57–63.

Management of behavioural problems in dementia

John Donoghue

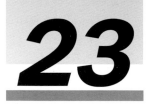

ZB, a 78-year-old woman lived until recently with her daughter and her family. Three years ago, she lived independently but since then has experienced slow progressive memory loss. She now cannot remember any recent events. She no longer wants to take part in any social activities, such as going out with the family. ZB frequently forgets things like putting on the kettle to boil water for tea. She has been asked not to attempt to cook meals and has had several disasters in the kitchen. Most recently, ZB has shown a distinct lack of personal hygiene.

Things have become particularly difficult over the last two months. ZB has become increasingly confused, agitated and verbally abusive to members of her family. Although she recognises her daughter, she thinks of her husband and children as strangers and is quite vehement in telling them to 'get out of this house'! ZB has also become increasingly suspicious of the family members, accusing them of stealing her money and personal effects. ZB's daughter is very worried about this and doesn't think it is safe for her mother to be left alone at home. She arranged for her to go into a private nursing home.

On admission to the nursing home, ZB became even more agitated and hostile and on two occasions assaulted members of staff when they tried to clean her after she had been incontinent. ZB started wandering at all times of the day and night and now gets only a few hours sleep.

The GP prescribed thioridazine 50 mg tds. ZB became drowsy, even more muddled, but somewhat easier to manage. A week after starting the thioridazine she fell while getting up from an easy chair and badly bruised her leg and arm. The GP has asked that she be admitted to hospital for assessment and advice about her treatment.

Her medication on admission was:

Ibuprofen	600 mg tds
Bendrofluazide	2.5 mg om
Vitamin capsules BPC	one tds
Thioridazine	50 mg tds and prn
Nitrazepam	5 mg nocte
Oxybutynin	2.5 mg tds

Her U and Es were normal, except for a sodium of 127 mmol/l (135–145, normal range). TFTs, FBC, LFTs and random glucose were normal.

ZB scored 6 out of 30 in a mini mental state examination. The working diagnosis was that of a dementing illness, probably of the Alzheimer's type.

Questions

1. Which aspects of this patient's behavioural problems are likely to be caused by her dementia, and which may have arisen from her management?
2. What alternative approaches are available to managing ZB?
3. What principles would you employ when considering drug treatment for this patient?

Note on Answers

Although there is currently a great deal of interest in developing medicines to prevent or delay cognitive decline in dementia, there are few data from controlled studies to support the use of medicines to manage behavioural problems. The answers below represent what is considered to be good practice. There is a paucity of good quality research in this patient group.

Answers

1. Which aspects of this patient's behavioural problems are likely to be caused by her dementia, and which may have arisen from her management?

Behavioural problems may occur as a consequence of the psychopathology of dementia, they may also occur as a result of poor or inappropriate management, or as a combination of these two factors.

A general decline in cognitive and visuo-spatial skills may render hazardous previously safe domestic and social activities. Difficulties with memory may cause frustration, anxiety and depression. Poor insight and judgement may mean that the patient attempts inappropriate or dangerous

activities or shows disregard for social norms of behaviour.

Underlying anxiety may be exacerbated by her removal from her familiar home environment, into the strange setting of the nursing home. Her cognitive impairment will make it extremely difficult for her to adapt to the new situation. Anxiety in dementia can present in different forms: emotional distress and agitation; physical symptoms such as headache, tachycardia, diarrhoea; and nuisance behaviour such as wandering or shouting.

Poor sleep can lead to maladaptive behaviour such as refusal to co-operate with staff, hostility and aggression. Confusion and inability to adapt may cause misinterpretation of other people's activities – for example, staff cleaning her after an episode of incontinence may be misinterpreted as an indecent assault and fiercely resisted. Persecutory ideas may emerge – a common one is accusing other people of theft when a patient cannot remember where they have left an item (often money).

There was a change in ZB's pattern of behaviour after being admitted to the nursing home. Her sleep deteriorated and she started wandering. This may have been a result of anxiety provoked by her inability to adapt to her new and unfamiliar surroundings. Poor sleep in its turn may produce more non-co-operative behaviours and hostility and aggression. It seems likely that the difficulties have arisen from a combination of the underlying illness, the change in circumstances, and inadequate management of that change.

ZB's drug regimen may have contributed to her presentation in many ways. ZB is prescribed a regular dose of Ibuprofen. The reasons for this prescription are unknown. Ibuprofen can cause fluid retention and it should be noted that ZB receives a diuretic. Carbamazepine, bendrofluazide and thioridazine can cause hyponatraemia albeit by different mechanisms. Psychotropic drugs are known to be an important cause of hyponatraemia in the mentally ill (McAskill and Taylor, 1997). One of the physical manifestations of hyponatraemia is confusion, and in the case of ZB this may lead to a delirium superimposed on a progressive dementing illness.

ZB also receives oxybutynin, presumably for urinary incontinence. Oxybutynin is an anticholinergic drug which is known to cross the blood-brain barrier and reports of oxybutynin-induced acute confusional states in patients with pre-existing cognitive impairment have been published (Donnellan et al, 1997).

ZB receives nitrazepam, a benzodiazepine hypnotic with a long half-life. Daytime drowsiness would be expected in an elderly person and this may contribute to cognitive impairment and falls.

Antipsychotics, such as thioridazine, are commonly prescribed in nursing homes for the elderly, primarily to control non-specific behaviours exhibited by patients with dementia. One survey in the UK found that 24% of nursing home residents were prescribed regular antipsychotics (McGrath and Jackson, 1996). This is despite the fact that specialist nurses and doctors working with dementia patients seem to have realistic expectations of the efficacy of this intervention (Thacker, 1997), that is, that it might not be beneficial.

If an antipsychotic is to be prescribed for ZB, thioridazine is probably not the best choice, though it is prescribed almost routinely in these situations.

Thioridazine is sedative, may cause postural hypotension and may also cause, because of its profound anticholinergic effects, cognitive impairment leading to acute confusional states. Sedating the patient may make her easier to manage, but may increase risks in other areas. There may be an increased risk of falls (Ray, 1992) with predictable sequelae. Indeed, falls are the main cause of accidental injuries in the elderly, and elderly females may be at higher risk of adverse sequelae because of the presence of osteoporosis. In dementia visuo-spatial co-ordination is often impaired, increasing risk of non-intentional injuries, and sedating drugs may exacerbate this. As already mentioned, drugs with a high anti-cholinergic load may hasten cognitive decline, making long term management even more problematic (McShane et al, 1997).

If antipsychotics are prescribed, the target behaviours should be described so that efficacy can be monitored. The threshold for such prescribing should be high and one should consider whether the behaviour places the individual or others at risk. The detailed review of this area published by the American Psychiatric Association (1997) is highly recommended.

2. What alternative approaches are available to managing ZB?

Many pharmacological strategies have been used to reduce the many non-specific behaviours seen in dementia patients. Such behaviours are difficult to measure and change in quality and quantity as the illness progresses. Controlled trials are virtually non-existent, but case studies and case series abound. These reports should be interpreted with caution.

In addition to antipsychotics, beta-blockers, buspirone, dexamphetamine, selegiline, carbamazepine, lithium, serotonergic antidepressants and chlormethiazole have all been claimed to be effective (Schneider and Sobin, 1991; Paton and Branford, 1997). These drugs should not be used before consultation of the primary literature. Such treatments should be closely monitored from both an efficacy and toxicity perspective. Whenever possible, however, the use of drugs to manage behavioural difficulties in dementia should be avoided. What many patients need is reassurance – given frequently – and to be distracted from inappropriate behaviours. Patients who wander often need reassurance that they are not 'lost'. Providing then with familiar personal objects may help. They also need to be provided with activities to prevent boredom. Some drugs may stimulate – for example, sympathomimetics, SSRI antidepressants and drinks containing caffeine. These should be avoided if they are thought to be a contributing factor.

Frustration at not being able to cope with activities of daily living can be reduced by dividing tasks into small, simple steps, with enough time allowed for completion. For example, it may take a demented person an hour to dress. Give repeated simple instructions and reassurance.

Suspiciousness and persecutory ideas may develop from forgetfulness. Take concerns seriously and offer help in looking for missing items. Encourage social interactions and do not be confrontational, even when objects have been 'stolen' on many occasions previously.

Incontinence should always be investigated for a possible physical cause. Where none is apparent, ensure that the patient is reminded frequently of the need to go to the toilet, or take them to the toilet regularly. Reduce or discontinue diuretics where possible, especially long-acting drugs and give only small amounts for bedtime drinks.

Poor sleep is often a problem in dementia. Give reassurance to alleviate anxiety. Avoid stimulating drinks or medicines at bedtime. Daytime activities can be increased to help ensure the patient is tired, and daytime sleeping should be discouraged. Physical problems, such as pain or hunger, should be considered and remedial action taken if necessary. A short-acting benzodiazepine or a chloral derivative may be helpful. Antipsychotics are a treatment of last resort, as already mentioned, they may hasten cognitive decline (McShane et al, 1997). (The above suggestions are adapted from Wilcock, 1997.)

3. What principles would you employ when considering drug treatment for this patient?

Drug treatment should be based on criteria of safety, effectiveness and appropriateness. As few drugs as possible should be used, as it is more difficult to predict responses in the elderly largely because of pharmacokinetic changes, which in turn may fluctuate. The understanding of the pharmacology of each drug should be applied, to predict potential therapeutic effects, adverse events and drug interactions.

Avoid changing more than one drug at a time, otherwise it is impossible to attribute either the response or any side effects which occur. Give drugs time to work. Psychotropic medicines may take longer to work in the elderly. For example, antidepressants may take as long as 8 weeks to provide any benefit (Georgotas et al, 1989).

Start treatment at low doses and increase doses only slowly. This will reduce the incidence of side effects and may allow responses at lower doses to emerge. For example, demented patients with psychotic symptoms may respond to doses of 1–2 mg/day of risperidone (Lee et al, 1994).

Select drugs with minimal effects in the following areas:
- anticholinergic
- sedative
- potential for postural hypotension

Lastly, avoid changing medication at critical points – for example, when transferring to another ward, or at discharge.

Key points

- The elderly are more prone to adverse drug reactions.
- Drugs with anticholinergic effects can cause delirium.
- If at all possible, the use of drugs to manage behavioural problems in dementia should be avoided.
- Antipsychotics are commonly prescribed to treat non-specific behaviours in dementia, despite a paucity of evidence to support their efficacy, and a significant side-effect profile.
- Other pharmacological strategies have been employed, but are poorly supported by objective evidence of efficacy.

References

American Psychiatric Association (1997) Practice Guideline for the treatment of patients with Alzheimer's disease and other dementias of late life, *Am J Psych* **154:** (5 Suppl), 1–39.

Donnellan CA, Food L, McDonald P (1997) Oxybutynin and cognitive dysfunction, *Br Med J* **315:** 1363–4.

Georgotas A, McCue E, Cooper TB (1989) A placebo-controlled comparison of nortriptyline and phenelzine in maintenance therapy of elderly depressed patients, *Arch Gen Psych* **46:** 783–6.

Lee H, Cooney JM, Lawlor BA (1994) The use of risperidone, an atypical neuroleptic, in Lewy body disease, *Int J Geriatric Psych* **9:** 415–17.

McAskill R, Taylor D (1997) Psychotropics and hyponatraemia, *Psych Bull* **21:** 33–5.

McGrath AM, Jackson GA (1996) Survey of neuroleptic prescribing in residents of nursing homes in Glasgow, *Br Med J* **312:** 611–12.

McShane R, Keene J, Gedling K et al (1997) Do neuroleptic drugs hasten cognitive decline in dementia? Prospective study with necropsy follow up, *Br Med J* **314:** 266–70.

Paton C, Dranford D (1997) Advances in the treatment of Alzheimer's disease, *Pharm J* **259:** 693–6.

Ray W (1992) Psychotropic drugs and injuries among the elderly: a review, *J Clin Psychopharmcol* **12:** 386–96.

Schneider LS, Sobin PB (1991) Non-neuroleptic medications in the management of agitation in Alzheimer's disease and other dementia: a selective review, *Int J Geriatric Psych* **6:** 691–708.

Thacker S (1997) Nurses' and doctors' expectations towards neuroleptic response in dementia, *Psych Bull* **21:** 670–2.

Wilcock GK (1997) Pharmacological and non-pharmacological therapeutic interventions in Alzheimer's disease, *Clinician* **15:**(1) 30–7.

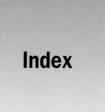

Index